Contents

COVENTRY UNIVERSITY
NURSING & MIDWIFERY LIBRARY

KU-184-857

3. Cardiac output studies   33

4. Patient case studies   55

Lanchester Library

LANCHESTER LIBRARY

3 8001 00211 3896

£10.95

24 AN
DIL
31563

Haemodynamic Profiles
and the
Critically Ill Patient

COVENTRY UNIVERSITY
NURSING & MIDWIFERY LIBRARY

Haemodynamic Profiles and the Critically Ill Patient

a practical guide

A. Dillon
Senior Clinical Nurse, General Intensive Care,
Queen Alexandra Hospital, Portsmouth, UK

J. Lyon
Lecturer Practitioner, University of Southampton School of
Nursing and Midwifery, Cardiothoracic Unit,
Southampton General Hospital, Southampton, UK

M.A. Coombs
Senior Nurse/SDU Manager, Intensive Care Unit,
John Radcliffe Hospital, Oxford, UK

Consultant Editors
T.M. Craft
Royal United Hospital, Bath, UK

R. Schneider
John Radcliffe Hospital, Oxford, UK

Lanchester Library

WITHDRAWN

3 8001 00211 3896

616 · 1028

βIOS
SCIENTIFIC
PUBLISHERS

© **BIOS Scientific Publishers Limited, 1997**

First published 1997

All rights reserved. No part of this book may be reproduced or transmitted, in any form or by any means, without permission.

A CIP catalogue record for this book is available from the British Library.

ISBN 1 859962 30 0

BIOS Scientific Publishers Ltd
9 Newtec Place, Magdalen Road, Oxford OX4 IRE, UK.
Tel. +44 (0)1865 726286. Fax +44 (0)1865 246823
World Wide Web home page: http://www.Bookshop.co.uk/BIOS/

To
friendship, family
and PRB

Important Note from the Publisher

The information contained within this book was obtained by BIOS Scientific Publishers Ltd from sources believed by us to be reliable. However, while every effort has been made to ensure its accuracy, no responsibility for loss or injury whatsoever occasioned to any person acting or refraining from action as a result of information contained herein can be accepted by the authors or publishers.

The reader should remember that medicine is a constantly evolving science and while the authors and publishers have ensured that all dosages, applications and practices are based on current indications, there may be specific practices which differ between communities. You should always follow the guidelines laid down by the manufacturers of specific products and the relevant authorities in the country in which you are practising.

PO 488
16 / 1 /97

Typeset by Florencetype Ltd, Stoodleigh, Tiverton, Devon, UK.
Printed by Biddles Ltd, Guildford, UK.

Coventry University

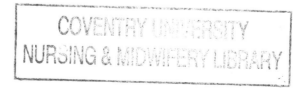
COVENTRY UNIVERSITY
NURSING & MIDWIFERY LIBRARY

Abbreviations

A&E	accident and emergency
AaDO$_2$	alveolar–arterial oxygen difference
ALI	acute lung injury
ARDS	adult respiratory distress syndrome
AV	atrioventricular
AvDO$_2$	arteriovenous oxygen difference
BP	blood pressure
BSA	body surface area
cAMP	cyclic adenosine monophosphate
CaO$_2$	arterial oxygen content
CI	cardiac index
CO	cardiac output
CPB	cardiopulmonary bypass
CvO$_2$	venous oxygen content
CVP	central venous pressure
Cx	circumflex branch
DO$_2$	oxygen delivery
DO$_2$I	oxygen delivery index
ECG	electrocardiogram
ECMO	extra corporeal membrane oxygenation
EDV	end-diastolic volume
FG	French gauge
FIO$_2$	fraction of inspired oxygen
Hb	haemoglobin
HR	heart rate
ICU	intensive care unit
IVC	inferior vena cava
L(R)CWI	left (right) cardiac work index
L(R)VSWI	left (right) ventricular stroke work index
LA	left atrium
LAD	left anterior descending
LCA	left coronary artery
LV	left ventricle
LVAD	left ventricular assist device
LVEDP	left ventricular end-diastolic pressure
MAP	mean arterial pressure
MV	mitral valve

O_2AV	oxygen availability
O_2AVI	oxygen availability index
PA	pulmonary artery
Pa	pulmonary alveolar
PaO_2	partial pressure of arterial oxygen
PADP	pulmonary artery diastolic pressure
PAP	PA pressure
PAWP	PA wedge pressure
PB	barometric pressure
PEEP	positive end-expiratory pressure
pHi	intramucosal pH
PV	pulmonary valve
Pv	pulmonary venous
PVR	pulmonary vascular resistance
RA	right atrium
RAP	right atrial pressure
RCA	right coronary artery
RV	right ventricle
RVAD	right ventricular assist device
RVEDV	right ventricular end-diastolic volume
RVEF	right ventricular ejection fraction
RVESV	right ventricular end-systolic volume
RVP	right ventricular pressure
RVSV	right ventricular stroke volume
SaO_2	saturation of arterial oxygen
SIRS	septic inflammatory response syndrome
SL	semilunar
SNS	sympathetic nervous system
SV	stroke volume
SVC	superior vena cava
SVI	stroke volume index
SvO_2	mixed venous oxygen saturation
SVR	systemic vascular resistance
SVRI	systemic vascular resistance index
TV	tricuspid valve
VO_2	oxygen consumption
VO_2I	oxygen consumption index
VSD	ventricular septal defect

Preface

The original idea for this book came from experience of using pulmonary artery catheters and from the questions that arose from practice.

The aim of this book is to provide easily accessible information that can be used at the bedside by all health care professionals in contact with patients requiring haemodynamic monitoring.

We anticipate that readers will have some basic knowledge and skills in managing a patient with a pulmonary artery catheter, but may not have an in-depth understanding of the rationale underpinning their use. The information provided will assist in directing practice actions. It is envisaged that greater understanding of this area will result from application of this knowledge in practice. The book is planned as a practical guide with summary notes and highlighted practice points to inform on patient management.

The book is intended to provide immediate access to useful clinical information in the form of a pocket guide for practitioners. It is not intended to give a detailed, in-depth review. For this reason, references mentioned are included in the further reading sections at the end of each chapter.

A. Dillon
J. Lyon
M.A. Coombs

CHAPTER 1

Overview of Cardiac Anatomy and Physiology

1. INTRODUCTION

This chapter reviews aspects of cardiac anatomy and physiology relevant to the interpretation of cardiac output studies and cardiac function.

2. FUNCTION

To maintain a stable state at cellular and organ level, the cardiovascular system adjusts to the demands of tissues. This involves:

- the transport of oxygen, glucose and hormones to all body tissues;
- the removal of metabolic end-products from the tissues for break-down and elimination;
- the redistribution of heat energy from active tissue.

The cardiovascular system comprises two major sub-systems: pulmonary circulation and systemic circulation. The pulmonary circulation is supplied by blood from the right side of the heart and brings desaturated blood into close proximity with oxygen-rich air before returning it to the left side of the heart. The systemic circulation is supplied with oxygenated blood from the left side of the heart and supplies the body with oxygen and nutrients before returning the deoxygenated blood to the right side of the heart.

3. DESCRIPTION AND LOCATION

The heart is a hollow, cone-shaped, muscular pump weighing approximately 340 g (*Figure 1*). The average adult heart is 14 cm long and 9 cm wide at its base. Situated in the mediastinum, the heart lies obliquely between the lungs and is bordered by the spine and sternum. Two-thirds of the heart extends left of the midline. The base lies beneath the second rib and extends downwards and to the left. The apex (tip) terminates at the fifth intercostal space.

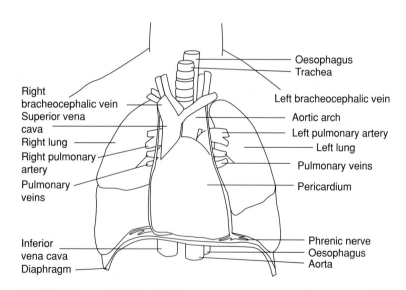

Figure 1. The thoracic cavity and contents.

PRACTICE POINT

To detect the apical heartbeat, auscultate between ribs 5 and 6, 7.5 cm to left of the midline (for normal build).

---

4. ANATOMY

4.1 Cardiac chambers

The heart is divided into four chambers which can be seen functionally as two separate systems: the **right heart** and the **left heart** (*Figure* 2).

The **right heart** is composed of the **right atrium** (RA) and the **right ventricle** (RV), which are separated by the **tricuspid valve** (TV). Deoxygenated blood is received from the body into the RA and pumped by the RV via the **pulmonary valve** (PV) into the low-pressure pulmonary circulation.

The **left heart** is composed of the **left atrium** (LA) and **left ventricle** (LV), which are separated by the **mitral valve** (MV). Oxygenated blood is received from the lungs and pumped by the LV via the **aortic valve** into the high-pressure systemic circulation.

The septum, valves and support structures are formed from connective tissue. The right and left heart are divided by the interatrial septum and a thicker interventricular septum. Following closure of the foramen ovale after birth, there should be no connections between the left and right side of the heart.

The RA has a smooth-walled posterior and a rough anterior part and the openings of the superior and inferior venae cavae are guarded by rudimentary valve structures. The RV is divided into an inflow portion near the tricuspid valve (main body) and the outflow tract (infundibulum). Separating these is a muscular ridge, the infundibulo-ventricular crest. The inner aspect of the inflow tract is rough and contains the origins of the papillary muscles. The outflow tract is smooth-walled and directed upwards towards the right pulmonary trunk. The right ventricular cavity is crescent-shaped and has a 'bellow'-like pumping action.

The LA is smaller than the RA but has thicker walls. The four pulmonary veins enter on the upper posterior wall and the fossa ovalis depression is on the septal surface. The main part of the cavity is smooth.

The LV (except the fibrous vestibule below the aortic orifice) is marked by thick trabeculae. The cavity of the LV is cone-shaped and contraction of the ventricle occurs at the apex and progresses towards the base in a spiral fashion. The openings of the right and left coronary arteries are in the sinuses of the Valsalva which are proximal to the aortic valve.

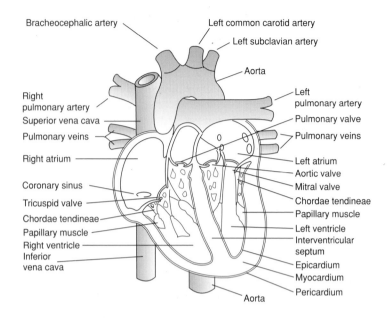

Figure 2. Structure of the heart.

4.2 Heart wall

The heart is enveloped in a three-layered sac called the pericardium. The outer layer is the **parietal pericardium**; this is fibrous and fatty, and is attached to the proximal ends of the large blood vessels, the diaphragm, the back of the sternum and the vertebrae to provide anchorage. At the origin of the aortic arch, the parietal pericardium is reflected back to form the serous **visceral pericardium (epicardium)**. This contains blood vessels, lymph capillaries and nerve fibres. Deeper portions contain fat along the paths of larger coronary vessels. Between the parietal and visceral pericardium exists a potential space, the pericardial cavity, which has a small amount of serous fluid acting to reduce friction during cardiac movement.

The relatively thick middle layer is the **myocardium**, composed of cardiac muscle. It is arranged in planes separated by connective tissue, with a rich blood and lymph supply. Heart wall thickness varies throughout: the atrial wall is 2–3 mm; the RV wall is 2–5 mm; and the LV 12–15 mm to generate higher pressures to overcome systematic resistance. The myocardial tissue is composed of both contractile and conducting elements. The muscle fibres form complex figure-of-eight spirals, creating a syncytium of fibres. The presence of the intercalated discs creates an interconnected branching network with low electrical resistance, allowing electrical conduction and contraction.

The inner layer, the **endocardium**, consists of epithelial and connective tissue and collagenous/elastic fibres. The Purkinje fibres, important in cardiac conduction, are also located here. The endocardium lines all heart chambers and heart valves. It is continuous with the inner linings of blood vessels attached to the heart.

4.3 Heart valves

Heart valves are outgrowths of fibrous tissue which provide the entrance and exit from the cardiac chambers. They comprise the following:

- annulus – fibrous supporting ring,
- cusps – valve leaflets,
- chordae tendineae – supporting strands,
- papillary muscles – muscular columns,
- commissures – junctional areas between the valve cusps.

The **semilunar (SL) valves (pulmonary and aortic)** are situated between the ventricles and the major arteries. The SL valve structure is similar to that of the atrioventricular valves (AV), but above each leaflet of the aortic valve there is a small recess (the sinus of Valsalva) which holds and directs blood flow in coronary filling. During ventricular systole the valve cusps are forced open against the arterial wall, allowing blood to flow through. As blood flow slows, small circular currents are generated in the spaces between the arterial wall and the valve cusps, which close the cusps.

The **atrioventricular (AV) valves (mitral and tricuspid)** are situated between the atria and ventricles. During diastole, the AV valves open passively owing to the lower pressure in the ventricles. At end-diastole, the pressure in the ventricles increases, assisting AV valve closure. The valve cusps are kept in position by contraction of the papillary muscles and tension from the chordae tendineae.

Damage to heart valves can result in stenosis or regurgitation. Stenosis increases the pressures required to move the blood through the valve; regurgitation will occur through an incompetent valve. Any turbulent blood flow across an abnormal valve will produce a murmur.

4.4 Great vessels

The RA receives blood from the superior vena cava (SVC), the inferior vena cava (IVC) and the coronary sinus. The small Thebesian veins drain small amounts of blood directly from the atrial wall into both right and left atria. The oxygen saturation of blood returning to the heart varies; 80% in the IVC; 70% in the SVC; and 30% in the cardiac veins, the last value resulting from the high rate of extraction of oxygen by the cardiac muscle.

PRACTICE POINT

Owing to these differences, true mixed venous O_2 saturation sampling can only be obtained in the pulmonary artery (PA). A normal mixed venous O_2 saturation is 75%.

Blood is directed through the right side of the heart to the main pulmonary trunk. This divides into the left and right pulmonary arteries to the lungs. Blood is returned to the heart via the four pulmonary veins, emptying into the LA. The blood moves through the left side of the heart and is ejected into the ascending aorta. It is then distributed to the coronary arteries, the arch of the aorta and into the thoracic and the abdominal aorta.

4.5 Coronary arteries

The coronary arteries arise from the aorta, just beyond the aortic valve. They spread over the epicardial surface, branching from the epicardium to the myocardium and on to the endocardium.

There are two main coronary arteries. The **right coronary artery** (RCA) leaves the aorta from the anterior surface and descends diagonally between the RA and RV in the atrioventricular groove. The RCA divides into:

- the marginal artery, supplying the anterior, lateral and posterior areas of the RV; and
- the posterior descending artery, supplying the posterior wall of both the RV and LV and the posterior ventricular septum.

The **left coronary artery** (LCA) leaves the aorta from the posterior surface and passes behind the PA. The LCA divides into:

- the left anterior descending (LAD), supplying the anterior and apical portion of the LV, the septum, papillary muscles, the bundle branches and the RV; and
- the circumflex (Cx), supplying the LA, the posterior LV and the papillary muscles.

Blood flow in the coronary circulation occurs predominantly in diastole, when there is reduced pressure generated in the myocardium. The continuous activity of the cardiac tissue requires a constant supply of oxygen and nutrients. As only one-twentieth of the cardiac output (CO) flows through the coronary arteries, there needs to be maximal oxygen extraction.

4.6 Coronary veins

Deoxygenated blood is returned to the RA by a large coronary sinus. There are two main coronary veins; the **great cardiac vein** drains the anterior aspect, and the **middle cardiac vein** drains the posterior aspect of the heart.

5. PHYSIOLOGY

5.1 Cardiac cycle

Systole refers to the phase of contraction and diastole to the phase of relaxation. The cardiac cycle (*Figure 3*) is the period from one contraction to the next; it lasts approximately 0.8 sec, depending on heart rate. During the cardiac cycle, blood continuously flows from the IVC/SVC and coronary sinus to the RA, and from the pulmonary veins into the LA. Approximately 70% of blood flows passively into the ventricles prior to atrial contraction. As atrial pressure increases, blood is pushed into the ventricle through the open AV valve. This remains open as long as atrial pressure is higher than the pressure in the relaxed ventricle. The blood enters the ventricle, but cannot leave because of the closed SL valve.

> **PRACTICE POINT**
> Synchronous atrial contraction contributes 20% of ventricular filling; loss of this 'atrial kick' can be detrimental to stroke volume and therefore CO. If blood pressure suddenly drops, analyse cardiac rhythm to see if sinus rhythm has been lost.

As the ventricles contract, the pressure builds up rapidly and causes closure of the AV valves (first heart sound). The pressure continues to rise rapidly against the closed valves. This is the period of **isovolumetric ventricular contraction**, which lasts approximately 0.05 sec. When ventricular pressure exceeds arterial pressure, the SL valves open and blood is ejected into the arteries. This is **ventricular ejection**. The ventricular pressure then begins to fall below arterial pressure and the SL valves close (second heart sound). Approximately 60% of the blood is ejected by the ventricle; this is referred to as the **ejection fraction**.

As the AV valves are closed, no blood enters or leaves the ventricles. As the muscles relax, the pressure in the ventricles falls. This is known as **isovolumetric ventricular relaxation**. When ventricular pressure is less

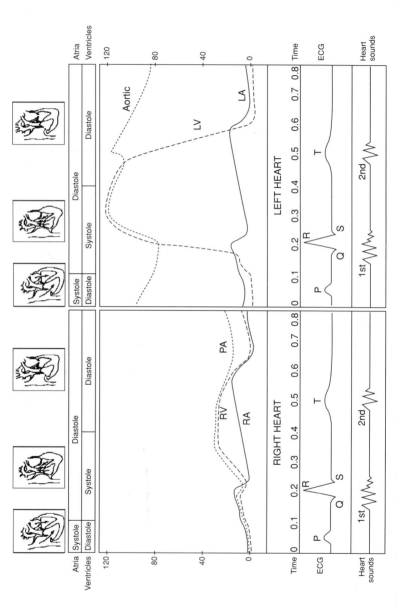

Figure 3. The cardiac cycle. Modified from Tortora and Anagnostakos, *Principles of Anatomy and Physiology*, 4th Edn, p. 469.
Published by Harper & Row, New York.

than the atrial pressure, the AV valves open and the SL valves close. The closing of the SL valves produces a brief rise in arterial pressure (dicrotic notch) and the second heart sound. Blood continues to enter the atria causing increased pressure. When this becomes greater than ventricular pressure, the AV valves open and blood flows into the ventricles (**ventricular filling**).

5.2 Preload

The circulation of the blood is maintained by the effective pumping action of the heart. The volume of blood delivered will vary depending on metabolic rate and on altered physiology, caused, for example, by exercise, sleep, age, emotional stress or pregnancy. **Preload** refers to the presystolic or end-diastolic length of the myocardial fibre. Work performed by Otto Frank and Ernest Starling demonstrated that increasing the length of the myocardial fibre prior to contraction results in an increased contraction and stroke volume. This is known as the **Frank–Starling Law** (*Figure 4*). In practical terms, increasing filling pressures by administering volume can increase stroke volume and therefore cardiac output.

PRACTICE POINT

Patients with cardiac failure may need higher filling pressures with volume loading to generate an increased CO. Careful volume challenges with close monitoring of the right- and left-side cardiac pressures will help determine the optimum filling parameters.

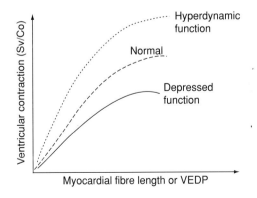

Figure 4. Frank–Starling curve.

5.3 Contractility

The strength of cardiac contraction reflects the speed of myocardial fibre shortening. It is largely independent of preload and is achieved by stimulation of the sympathetic nervous system (SNS). Decreased cardiac contractility can be caused by acidosis, hypoxaemia, hypokaleamia, drug toxicity or infection.

5.4 Compliance

Compliance is the rate of change in ventricular volume compared to the change in diastolic pressure (*Figure 5*). In a healthy heart, volume administration does not cause a dramatic rise in end-diastolic pressure – the ventricle is compliant. In certain disease states (e.g. pericardial effusion/ tamponade, cardiac failure and cardiomyopathies) the ventricle is less compliant and 'stiff', and administering volume can cause a dramatic rise in end-diastolic pressure.

> **PRACTICE POINT**
> Any patient considered to have decreased compliance will need careful fluid challenges. A broad guide is to give 200 ml colloid over 10 min. Repeat cardiovascular assessment 5 min later. If filling pressures do not rise by 3 mmHg and the wedge pressure remains acceptable, then further volume can be given.

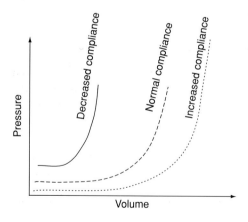

Figure 5. Compliance curve.

5.5 Afterload

Afterload is the resistance that the ventricles must pump against when ejecting blood. Pressure is the product of flow and resistance. If resistance in the system is high, blood flow will decrease unless the pressure generated also increases.

Increased LV afterload is determined by the pressure in the aorta, the systemic vascular resistance (SVR), and the volume and viscosity of blood in the aorta. It can be affected by sepsis which alters the SVR. RV afterload is determined by the pressure in the pulmonary system and may be increased by pulmonary hypertension, pulmonary embolus or acidosis.

5.6 Cardiac output

Cardiac output (CO) is the amount of blood ejected from the left ventricle into the aorta each minute. It is determined by stroke volume (SV) and heart rate (HR).

6. THE NERVOUS SYSTEM

6.1 Sympathetic nervous system (SNS)

The SNS is activated during times of stress. It is regulated by the vasomotor centre through peripheral sympathetic fibres and secretion of adrenaline and noradrenaline from the adrenal medulla. SNS stimulation produces the 'flight or fight' response, with resultant tachycardia, increased cardiac contractility and peripheral vasoconstriction. Tissues and organs innervated by the SNS contain type-specific receptors which can be targeted with drugs. The classification of adrenoreceptors is shown in *Table 1*.

6.2 Parasympathetic nervous system

Fibres from the parasympathetic nervous system to the heart are contained within the vagus nerve. These fibres are almost exclusively in the atria, and vagal stimulation causes a reduction in heart rate. Some vagal fibres may be present in the ventricles and stimulation of these may cause a reduction in cardiac contractility.

The baroreceptors are located in the walls of the carotid sinuses and in the aortic arch. These pressure receptors are stimulated by changes in the patient's blood pressure; they transmit signals to the vasomotor centre in the medulla, effecting an appropriate response in the arterial blood pressure.

Table 1. Classification of adrenoceptors

Type	Site	Effect of stimulation
α_1	Skin and mucosa	Arterial vasoconstriction (including renal/mesenteric)
	Ventricles	Increased contractility
α_2	Veins	Vasoconstriction
		Feedback inhibition of noradrenaline
β_1	SA node	Increased rate
	Atrial muscle	Increased contractility
	AV node	Increased conduction
	Ventricles	Increased contractility
β_2	Bronchial smooth muscle	Relaxation
	Veins	Vasodilatation (including renal/ mesenteric)
	Dopaminergic	Dilation of splanchnic and renal vascular smooth muscle

7. FURTHER READING

Guyton, A. (1991) *Textbook of Medical Physiology.* W.B. Saunders, Philadelphia.

Little, R.C. (1985) *Physiology of the Heart and Circulation,* 3rd Edn. Year Book Medical Publishers, Chicago.

Sanderson, R. and Kurth, C. (1983) *The Cardiac Patient: a Comprehensive Approach,* 2nd Edn. W.B. Saunders, Philadelphia.

Sarnoff, S.J. (1955) Myocardial contractility as described by ventricular function curves. *Physiology Review,* **35**, 107–122.

Starling, E.H. (1918) *The Linacre Lecture on the Law of the Heart.* Longmans Green, London.

Tortora, G. and Anagnostakos, N. (1990) *Principles of Anatomy and Physiology.* Harpe International Editions, New York.

Underhill, S., Woods, S., Froelicher, E. and Halpenny, C. (1989) *Cardiac Nursing,* 2nd Edn. J.B. Lippincott, Philadelphia.

CHAPTER 2

Pulmonary Artery Catheters

I. INTRODUCTION

Haemodynamic monitoring with pulmonary artery (PA) catheters is used in the assessment of critically ill patients. It involves the frequent or continuous observation of cardiac, pulmonary and vascular parameters.

The first use of central venous pressure (CVP) monitoring was in 1962. However, the use of right-sided pressure monitoring to reflect left ventricular filling pressures in patients with serious cardiovascular disease may produce an inaccurate assessment of left ventricular function. An immediate and reliable means of assessing left ventricular function is vital in the management of the critically ill patient. In 1970, H.J.C. Swan and W. Ganz developed the balloon-tipped, flow-directed PA catheter to assist in the assessment of left ventricular function.

Despite the sophistication of available catheters, the benefit to the patient only comes from the knowledge and skill of the practitioner in utilizing the information gained. PA monitoring is only part of the assessment and the total needs of the patient must be recognized and built into a comprehensive care plan.

2. DESCRIPTION

2.1 Types of catheter

The adult PA catheter is:

- 7 French gauge (FG) – available in the range from 4.0 to 7.5 FG,
- 110 cm long (available from 60 cm to 110 cm in length),
- made from polyvinylchloride or polyurethane, pliable at body temperature,
- thromboresistant and kink resistant,
- radio-opaque with single narrow black markings at 10 cm and wide black markings at 50 cm.

The following types of PA catheter are available.

- The **fibre-optic PA catheter** is capable of continuously monitoring mixed venous oxygen saturation (SvO_2) for patients who demonstrate oxygen transport problems (delivery or consumption).
- The **sequential pacing catheter** has an electrode channel containing two ventricular and three atrial electrodes. This allows the catheter to monitor cardiac rhythm and enables atrial, ventricular and atrio-ventricular sequential pacing. It can be used in patients with cardiac dysrhythmias who need a PA catheter for cardiac assessment.

PRACTICE POINT

The pacing threshold with this catheter may be higher than with a standard pacing wire, with pacing thresholds in the ventricle requiring 4–5 milliamps.

- The **quadruple lumen catheter**, the standard type of PA catheter, provides basic left ventricular function assessment (*Figures 6* and *7*). This monitors RA pressure, PA pressure (PAP) and pulmonary artery wedge pressure (PAWP), and cardiac output (CO). The additional side port allows infusion of solutions without interfering with pressure monitoring. This catheter has four lumens.

  (i) The **distal lumen** ends at the tip of the catheter; PAP is measured and mixed venous blood samples are taken from this port. During insertion, chamber pressures can be monitored and measured as the catheter is floated through the heart.

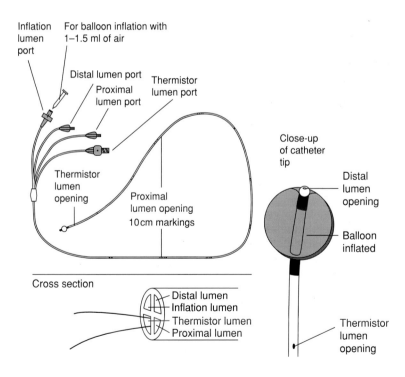

Figure 6. The quadruple lumen PA catheter.

COVENTRY UNIVERSITY
NURSING & MIDWIFERY LIBRARY

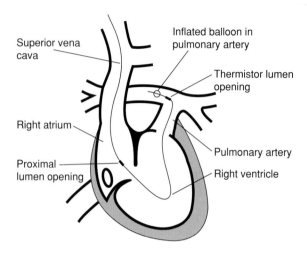

Figure 7. The quadruple lumen PA catheter *in situ* (right side of heart).

(ii) The **proximal lumen** opens at 30 cm from the tip and is used for injectate administration in CO calculation. RA pressures can be monitored and measured from this port.

(iii) The **thermistor lumen** contains electrical leads positioned on the catheter surface to detect temperature changes used to determine CO. It is located 4 cm from the catheter tip to reduce thermistor contact with the pulmonary vessel wall, thus preventing erroneously high CO readings.

(iv) The balloon **inflation lumen** is used to inflate and deflate the balloon with air during catheter insertion and PAWP measurement. Balloon capacity varies with size: 7 FG has a capacity of 1.5 ml and 5 FG a capacity of 0.8 ml. Balloon rupture will occur at approximately 3 ml. Water or saline should never be used as adequate deflation may be problematic and the excess weight can obstruct the flotation of the balloon. To reduce ectopic activity and valvular damage during catheter insertion, the balloon should be fully inflated.

3. INDICATIONS FOR USE

Pulmonary artery catheters are primarily used to obtain accurate information on both right and left heart pressures and function. Clinical guidelines are given in *Table 2*.

Table 2. Clinical guidelines

Assessment of cardiovascular function:
  Large myocardial infarction
  Cardiogenic shock
  Right ventricular infarction
  Cardiac tamponade
  Infusions of high dose vasoactive drugs
  Peri-operative monitoring of high-risk patients

Assessment of respiratory function:
  Cardiogenic or non-cardiogenic pulmonary oedema
  Adult respiratory distress syndrome (ARDS)
  Acute respiratory disease
  Pulmonary hypertension

Assessment of fluid requirements:
  Multiple trauma
  Multi-organ failure
  Extensive burns
  Sepsis

4. CATHETER INSERTION

The information given to the patient, family and friends must be easily understood, comprehensive and appropriate to needs. Often the patient is too sick or sedated to understand complex information. However, unconscious or sedated patients also need explanations regarding procedures. These explanations are vital in ensuring patient co-operation and in reducing patient anxiety.

4.1 Equipment preparation

The PA catheter can be inserted at the bedside 'blind', under fluoroscopy or in a cardiac catheter laboratory. The equipment required for catheter insertion is listed in *Table 3*.

Prior to insertion, a defibrillator and antiarrhythmic drugs should be readily available. Serum potassium and clotting should be checked and corrected if abnormal. Preoxygenation may be required in patients with impaired gas exchange. In hypovolaemia, volume replacement can aid flotation of the PA catheter through the heart. Any change of essential infusions should be planned prior to line insertion in order to minimize any disruption and potential problems to the patient.

Table 3. Equipment required for catheter insertion

Intravenous flush fluid +/− heparin, in accordance with unit protocol
Pressure bag
Transducer and monitoring tubing
Pressure monitoring modules
PA catheter
Injectate coil (+/− ice − consult unit protocol)
Stopcocks
Local anaesthetic
Syringes (5/10 ml)
Needles − for injection of local anaesthetic and flushing/aspirating of
    catheter
Suture material
Dressing or insertion pack with sterile drapes
Cleaning agent
Gloves/gowns and mask
Sedative agents as required
Chest X-ray form

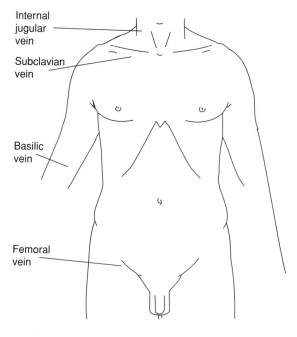

Internal jugular vein

Subclavian vein

Basilic vein

Femoral vein

Figure 8. Sites of insertion for pulmonary artery catheter.

4.2 Sites for insertion

The insertion sites for the PA catheter are shown in *Figure 8*. Advantages and disadvantages of the sites are listed in *Table 4*.

4.3 Procedural guidelines

- The ideal patient position is the Trendelenburg (head down), which produces venous engorgement and reduces risk of air entrainment. (This is not necessary if the femoral approach is used.)
- Accurate CO calculations require preprogrammed computer constants. Any changes in catheter size, injectate volume or temperature will need a different constant – details are usually supplied with the PA catheter.

Table 4. Advantages and disadvantages of insertion sites

Site	Advantages	Disadvantages
Internal jugular	Large vessel Easy to locate, easy access Short, straight path to SVC Low rate of complications	Uncomfortable for patient Close to carotid artery
Subclavian	Large vessel High flow rate Low infection rate Easy to maintain dressing Supra/infraclavicular approach Less restricting for patient	Risk of pneumothorax Close to subclavian artery Difficult to control bleeding Non-compressible vessel
Basilic	Accessible during resuscitation	Increased risk of phlebitis Increased time for drugs to circulation Catheter movement with arm Cut down approach
Femoral	Easy access Large vessel Accessible during resuscitation	Decreased patient mobility Increased rate of thrombosis Increased rate of infection Risk of femoral artery puncture Dressing problematic

---

PRACTICE POINTS
- No vasoactive drugs should be administered through the RA or PA port of the catheter; the side arm of the PA catheter can be used for fluids.
- With a femoral/brachial approach, the balloon should remain deflated until the catheter tip reaches a central thoracic vein. This is reflected in a marked deflection in the waveform baseline on patient coughing.

- The integrity of the balloon must be checked and the catheter flushed prior to insertion.
- The standard approach is via a percutaneous route. Following location and entry into the vein, a sheath introducer is inserted over a guide wire (the 'Seldinger' technique).
- As the catheter enters the RA, the balloon should be fully inflated. The RV should be reached after 30–40 cm as measured from the internal jugular site. Entry into the PA should occur no more than 20 cm from the RV. No more than 20 cm of catheter should be inserted without observing changes in the waveform (*Figure 9*).
- In patients with a large right atrium, low cardiac output or marked tricuspid incompetence, entrance of the catheter into the RV may prove problematic. In self-ventilating patients, a deep inspiration during advancement may prove useful.
- The electrocardiogram (ECG) monitor must be observed continuously for ectopic activity as the catheter comes into contact with the tricuspid valve and the endocardium of the RV.
- The resting position of the catheter (balloon deflated) will be in the left or right pulmonary artery. Following insertion, the balloon is reinflated to determine PAWP. The balloon is then deflated and the catheter returns to a PA position. The characteristic waveform should be displayed continuously.

4.4 Pressure waveforms: interpretation and analysis

Normal values of intracardiac pressure are given in *Table 5*.

Table 5. Normal intracardiac pressure values

Right atrial pressure (RAP)	2–6 mmHg
Right ventricular pressure (RVP)	25/0 mmHg
Pulmonary artery pressure (PAP)	25/8 mmHg
Pulmonary artery wedge pressure (PAWP)	8–12 mmHg

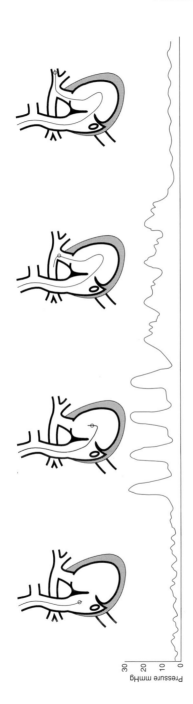

Pressure mmHg

Figure 9. Progression of the PA catheter through the heart showing the changes in waveform that should be observed.

Right atrial pressure waveform

The RAP waveform (*Figure 10*) has three positive waves, *a*, *c* and *v*, and three negative waves, *x*, *x¹* and *y*, where:

- *a* = increase in pressure during RA systole,
- *x* = descent representing atrial relaxation,
- *c* = increase of pressure due to ballooning of tricuspid valve (TV) during RV systole,
- *x¹* = atrioventricular movement during ventricular contraction,
- *v* = increase in pressure from atrial filling against closed TV,
- *y* = passive RA emptying after TV opening, before RA systole.

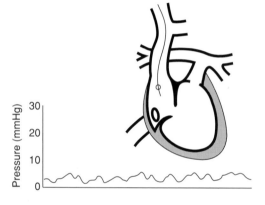

Figure 10. Right atrial pressure waveform.

PRACTICE POINT

Waveform analysis can indicate cardiac dysrhythmia; for example, if no *a* wave (RA contraction) is seen, this may indicate that the patient is in atrial fibrillation. The a wave may be larger in tricuspid stenosis because of the higher pressure needed to eject blood into the RV.

Right ventricular pressure waveform

The RVP waveform (*Figure 11*) is taller with sharp peaks resulting from higher ventricular systolic pressure generated during isovolumetric contraction. When RVP exceeds maximum PAP, the pulmonary valve opens, blood is ejected out of the RV, and the RVP drops quickly, resulting in lower diastolic pressures.

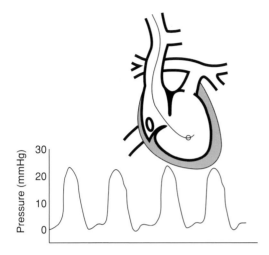

Figure 11. Right ventricular pressure waveform.

Pulmonary artery pressure waveform

PA systolic pressure should equal RV systolic pressure. The steep rise in PAP causes a sharp rise in the PAP waveform (*Figure 12*). When RVP falls below PAP, the pulmonary valve closes, causing a dicrotic notch on the downstroke of the waveform. The pressure generated by the blood against a closed pulmonary valve produces a diastolic pressure of 5–8 mmHg.

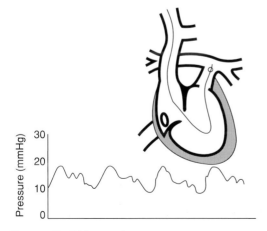

Figure 12. PAP waveform.

Pulmonary artery wedge pressure waveform

The waveform of the PAWP (*Figure 13*) is similar to the RAP waveform, with two to three positive waves (*a*, *c* and *v*) followed by negative waves (*x*, *y*), where:

 a = small rise in pressure due to atrial contraction,
 x = descent in pressure due to atrial relaxation,
 c = increase in pressure from mitral valve closure,
 v = increase due to atrial filling,
 y = descent due to rapid passive filling of LV from atria.

The PAWP is calculated as a mean of *a* and *v* waves which are usually of the same size.

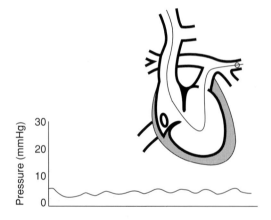

Figure 13. PAWP waveform.

PRACTICE POINT
Document pressures and observe waveforms during catheter placement. This will confirm the position of the catheter as it advances through the heart, and provide baseline information should the catheter become displaced at a later date.

---

5. COMPLICATIONS

A chest X-ray (anterior–posterior) should be taken immediately after insertion to ensure correct positioning of the PA catheter (*Figures 15* and *16*).

This will exclude any complications, for example pneumothorax, pleural effusion or tamponade. The catheter tip should lie in zone 3 of the lung, as classified by West (*Figure 14, Table 6*) to provide accurate information on left atrial pressures and not the higher reflected alveolar pressures.

A non-zone 3 position may be suspected if the wedge pressure increases by more than half the positive end-expiratory pressure (if the patient is ventilated) or if there is an excessive respiratory variation in the wedge trace.

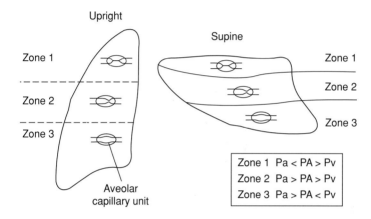

Figure 14. Zones of the lung, as classified by West. Reproduced from West, J. (1990) *Respiratory Physiology – The Essentials,* 4th Edn. With permission from Waverly, Baltimore, MD.

Table 6. Zones of the lung, and associated pressures

Zone	Position	Alveolar and vascular pressures
1	Found at tip of lung in upright position	Alveolar pressure is high
2	At level just above right atrium	Arterial pressure exceeds alveolar pressure
3	Gravity dependent area of lower lung	Greatest perfusion – arterial and left atrial pressures exceed alveolar pressure

With increased positive end-expiratory pressure (PEEP) or hypovolaemia, a larger portion of the lung may be converted to zone 1 or 2.

5.1 Cardiac dysrhythmias

Cardiac dysrhythmias occur if the unprotected catheter tip irritates the endocardium or the heart valves, particularly within the RV structures. Increased dysrhythmias may indicate displacement of the PA catheter. The PA catheter waveform must be monitored continuously and identified. The appearance of an RV waveform on the monitor will require refloating of the catheter.

5.2 Pulmonary infarction

If the balloon is left inflated or migrates into a pulmonary capillary for more than 15–20 sec, pulmonary infarction can occur. During the wedging procedure, the balloon should only be inflated for two to four respiratory cycles or under 15 sec. The PA waveform must be monitored and identified continuously.

5.3 Infection

It is essential to maintain aseptic techniques at all times. Early infections are due to poor aseptic technique during insertion. If the patient becomes pyrexial, full screening should be performed without delay. If infection is confirmed, the PA catheter must be removed.

The catheter must be properly secured to the patient so that non-sterile parts do not migrate and cause infection. Sterile caps must be used to cover all ports. The sterile plastic sleeve over the PA catheter allows repositioning of the catheter without compromising sterility.

5.4 Bleeding

Bleeding can be a problem in patients with clotting abnormalities. All catheter ports should be kept visible. The risk of accidental disconnection needs to be appreciated and managed appropriately in anxious or confused patients.

Figure 15. PA catheter – jugular approach and anatomical landmarks. 1a, PA catheter, right internal jugular. 1b, PA catheter, RA. 1c, PA catheter, MPA into PA. 2, CVP catheter, left internal jugular. 3, endotracheal tube. 4, left intercostal drain. 5, aortic arch/knuckle. 6, heart border. 7, costaphrenic angle. 8, diaphragm. 9, tricuspid valve. 10, pulmonary valve. 11, mitrial valve. 12 aortic valve. 13, lung shadowing secondary to adult respiratory distress syndrome.

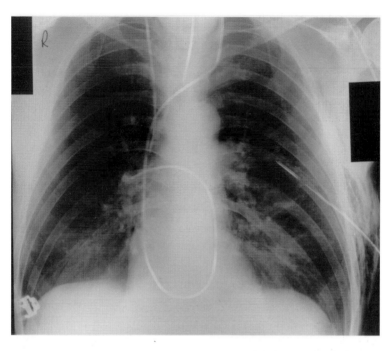

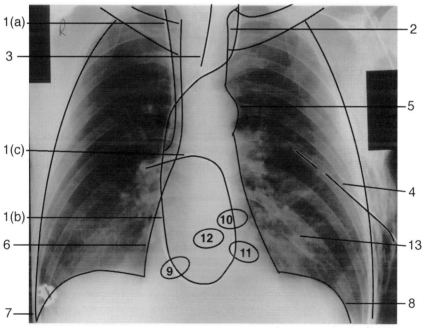

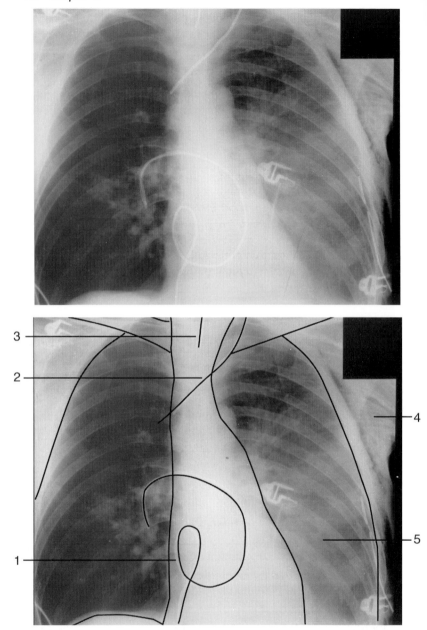

Figure 16. PA catheter – femoral approach. 1, hoop into RA, into MPA, into right RA. 2, CVP catheter, left internal jugular. 3, endotracheal tube. 4, surgical emphysema. 5, increased shadowing left mid and lower zone-consolidation.

5.5 Air embolism

Air embolism occurs if the balloon ruptures. Latex balloons absorb lipo-proteins from the blood and gradually lose their elasticity, causing balloon disintegration and rupture. Most PA balloons can withstand up to 72 inflations without rupturing. To reduce the risk of this and other complications, it is usual clinical practice to keep the catheter in place for up to 72 hours.

5.6 Pulmonary thromboembolism

Pulmonary thromboembolism results from thrombus formation and migration from the catheter. All traces of blood must be removed from the PA catheter, tubing and stopcocks following blood sampling. Catheter patency can be maintained by ensuring that the flushing device is used and maintained properly. If a femoral or brachial site has been used, the limb must be observed for ischaemia, vasospasm, oedema or inflammation indicating local venous obstruction.

5.7 Pulmonary artery rupture

PA rupture is caused by the catheter tip migrating through the PA wall or by over-inflation of the balloon, therefore only the recommended inflation volumes should be used. If less than the recommended amounts of air are used to wedge the balloon, the catheter may migrate; a chest X-ray will confirm catheter position.

> **PRACTICE POINT**
> If pulmonary artery diastolic pressure (PADP) correlates with PAWP, this can be used as a 'guide PAWP'.

5.8 Catheter kinking and intracardiac knotting

Catheter kinking is caused by the insertion of an excessive length of catheter. A guide to the distance from insertion site to the RA is given in *Table 7*. Knotting may be resolved by the use of a guidewire or, if unsuccessful, exploratory surgery.

6. PRACTITIONER RESPONSIBILITIES

The following guidelines should be used in association with unit protocol.

Table 7. Approximate measurement guide to RA

Insertion site	Distance to RA (cm)
Internal jugular/subclavian vein	35
Femoral vein	50
Right antecubital fossa	60
Left antecubital fossa	75

6.1 Documentation of recordings

The recommended frequency with which the given parameters should be measured is shown in *Table 8*.

Table 8. Parameters and frequency of measurement

Parameter	Frequency
Heart rate and rhythm	Hourly
Blood pressure (including mean aterial pressure)	Hourly
CVP	Hourly
PAP	Hourly
PAWP	On take-over of patient to determine baseline or on any change in clinical condition
CO studies	4–8 hourly or on any change in clinical condition or treatment
Core temperature	Hourly
Pressure bag	8 hourly, to check sufficient fluid and pressure
Zero transducers	8 hourly
Calibration of system	As per unit protocol

6.2 Equipment

Although most transducers are sufficiently sophisticated and have in-built safeguards against electrical damage, basic principles of electrical safety must be observed.

6.3 Patient care

Care and sleep periods must be planned to enable the patient to achieve maximum rest time. Information given to the patient, family or friends must be consistent and appropriate to their needs, and should provide a frame-work to enable understanding of the treatment plan and patient progress. Treatment and direction of care should come from an agreed team approach.

PRACTICE POINT

The PA transducer must be aligned to a zero reference point, for example patient's RA (phlebostatic axis – mid-axilla fourth intercostal space) or sternal notch. This must become the consistent baseline position for read-ings. A 1 cm drift in baseline produces a 0.8 mmHg difference in pressure measurements.

IMPORTANT POINTERS IN PATIENT CARE

* Care for the patient, not the catheter.
* Know why the patient has a PA catheter.
* Know and understand each drug administered; determine optimum treatment parameters (i.e. drug and fluid prescriptions).
* Aim to improve cardiac output/cardiac index through manipulation of preload and afterload and not just blood pressure.
* Do not manipulate preload, contractility and afterload together.
* Be proactive in your care.

7. CATHETER REMOVAL

The following information should act as a guideline only, and should be used in association with unit protocol. Throughout the procedure, the patient should be kept fully informed.

The following equipment is required:

* gloves,
* sterile gauze,
* dressing,
* suture cutter,
* sterile container for tip for microbiology screening.

These steps should be followed when removing a catheter.

(i) Ensure that there is adequate intravenous access prior to removal.
(ii) Check the most recent clotting results and correct any abnormali-ties before catheter removal.

(iii) Place patient in Trendelenburg position, if tolerated.

(iv) Make final check that the balloon is deflated.

(v) Using aseptic technique, withdraw the catheter, observing monitor for dysrhythmias. Aim for catheter exit at 90° angle to skin to avoid contamination of tip end. In theory, catheter removal should be timed with maximum positive intrathoracic pressure to prevent air entrainment; there is debate concerning this and therefore removal is in accordance with unit protocol.

(vi) Apply direct pressure to the site for 5–10 minutes and then observe site for complications.

8. FURTHER READING

Darovic,G. (1987) *Haemodynamic monitoring: Invasive and Non-invasive Clinical Application.* W.B. Saunders, Philadelphia.

Dossey. B., Guzzetta, C. and Kenner, C. (1992) *Critical Care Nursing: Body–Mind–Spirit*, 3rd Edn. J.B. Lippincott, Philadelphia.

Lake, C.L. (ed.) (1990) *Clinical Monitoring.* W.B. Saunders, Philadelphia.

Roundtree, W.D. (1991) Removal of pulmonary artery catheters by registered nurses: a study of safety and complications. *Focus Critical Care*, **18**, 313–315.

Shoemaker, W.C., Ayers, S. and Grenik, A. (1989) *Textbook of Critical Care,* 2nd Edn. W.B. Saunders, Philadelphia.

Swan, H.J.C., Ganz, W. and Forrester, J.S. (1970) Catherisation of the heart in man with use of flow directed balloon tipped catheter. *New England Journal of Medicine*, **283**, 447–451.

West, J. (1990) *Respiratory Physiology – The Essentials*, 4th Edn. Williams and Wilkins, Baltimore.

CHAPTER 3

Cardiac Output Studies

1. INTRODUCTION

This chapter outlines the measurement, calculation and interpretation of all the parameters that are considered within cardiac output studies. Parameters can be measured directly (palpated, monitored) or indirectly (derived, calculated) to give further information about cardiovascular and pulmonary function.

2. DIRECT MEASUREMENTS

There are a number of standard patient observations which should be monitored continuously and used to direct and evaluate patient treatment plans.

2.1 Heart rate

HR = 60–100/min in adults

Heart rate (HR) is used to calculate CO (HR × SV = CO). Bradycardia (HR < 60/min in adults) can indicate an athletic state, medication (e.g. digoxin, β-blockade), excessive parasympathetic activity or conduction defects.

Tachycardia (HR > 100/min in adults) can indicate a physiological response to exercise or stress (pain, anxiety, pyrexia, shock), excessive sympathetic activity, medication (e.g. isoprenaline) or conduction defects.

PRACTICE POINT

It is important to recognize the cardiac rhythm. For example, loss of atrial systole in atrial fibrillation can account for a 20% fall in CO and a resultant drop in blood pressure.

2.2 Arterial systolic and diastolic blood pressure

Systolic pressure = 100–140 mmHg (age-dependent)
Diastolic pressure = 60–90 mmHg (age-dependent)

Arterial systolic and diastolic blood pressure (BP) reflects the tension within blood vessels during the cardiac cycle. It can be measured with a sphygmomanometer or more accurately with an intra-arterial catheter.

Hypertension can be associated with age, anxiety, pain, arteriosclerosis and disease (e.g. phaeochromocytoma). Hypotension can be associated with intravascular fluid disturbances (e.g. cardiac failure or volume depletion).

2.3 Mean arterial pressure

Normal mean arterial pressure = 80–95 mmHg

Mean arterial pressure (MAP) represents the mean pressure in the vascular system throughout the cardiac cycle. It needs to be maintained to sustain coronary artery and tissue perfusion.

$$MAP = \frac{systolic\ pressure + (diastolic\ pressure \times 2)}{3}$$

Abnormal readings are associated with the same causes as described for BP.

2.4 Right atrial pressure

Normal right arterial pressure = 2–10 mmHg

Right atrial pressure (RAP) is also referred to as central venous pressure (CVP). It is measured via a central venous line or via the RA lumen of the PA catheter and provides information about RV filling and function. The measurements can be expressed in mmHg or cm of H_2O, depending on the system used. To convert mmHg to cm H_2O, multiply the value by 1.34.

An increased RAP may be caused by right ventricular failure, pulmonary hypertension, tricuspid stenosis or regurgitation. It can also reflect chronic left ventricular failure and volume overload due to an increase in 'back pressure' throughout the system. Cardiac tamponade will also cause the RAP to rise due to the general constrictive pressure of the pericardium on the heart.

A decreased RAP indicates hypovolaemia.

2.5 Pulmonary artery pressure

Systolic   = 15–25 mmHg
Diastolic = 8–15 mmHg
Mean   = 10–20 mmHg

This reading is measured via the distal lumen of the PA catheter. The PA systolic pressure reflects the pressure generated by the RV during systole. The PA diastolic pressure reflects the pressure generated against a closed pulmonary valve during RV diastole.

Increased PAP is associated with hypoxia, pulmonary hypertension, pulmonary embolism, volume overload, left ventricular failure, mitral stenosis and administration of vasoconstrictive agents.

Decreased PAP corresponds to volume depletion and use of pulmonary vasodilating agents.

2.6 Pulmonary artery wedge pressure

Normal mean = 6–12 mmHg

If there is no obstruction from the left side of the heart, PAWP reflects left ventricular end-diastolic pressure (LVEDP). This is an indication of **preload** and therefore left-sided filling pressures. If the pulmonary artery diastolic pressure (PADP) and PAWP are similar, wedging the PA catheter can be performed less frequently.

In patients with mitral valve stenosis, left atrial myxoma and pulmonary embolus, obstruction is likely to be present and PAWP will read higher. With mitral insufficiency, abnormally high readings will occur. The incompetent valve produces large regurgitant *v* waves during atrial filling/ventricular contraction. The *a* wave will more accurately reflect the LVEDP.

In severe LV hypertrophy, restrictive cardiomyopathy, aortic regurgitation and cardiac tamponade, the LVEDP may be elevated considerably owing to decreased ventricular compliance. Initially the PAWP may remain lower until lung compliance decreases.

In pulmonary vascular disease (e.g. pulmonary hypertension, cor pulmonale, pulmonary embolus and Eisenmenger's syndrome), there will be a greater discrepancy between PADP and PAWP.

> **PRACTICE POINT**
> The following three criteria should be used to confirm that the PAWP is being correctly monitored:
>
> - the characteristic waveform is continuously seen on the monitor,
> - PAWP is less than MAP,
> - blood withdrawn from the PA catheter whilst in the wedge position has an O_2 saturation comparable with the patient's PaO_2.

An increased PAWP can indicate left ventricular failure, volume overload, pulmonary oedema or mitral stenosis.

A decreased PAWP can indicate volume depletion or reflect a patient's response to diuretics/positive inotropic agents.

Practical guide to wedging the PA catheter

The patient's position for measurements should be flat or tilted up to 20° with the head up. The 90° lateral decubitus position can be used as long as the midsternum or fourth intercostal space anteriorly is used as a zero reference point.

Balloon inflation should occur slowly to allow for continuous monitoring of the PA pressure contour. When the characteristic wedge trace is obtained, no further inflation of the balloon should occur. Wedging should be kept to a minimum of two to four respiratory cycles or 15 sec. During the wedging procedure, no flushing of the system should occur.

If a wedge trace is obtained at a lower balloon volume (< 1.0 ml), catheter migration into a distal branch may have occurred. If increased volumes are needed and clarity of the waveform is lost, **overwedging** has occurred. This reflects the pressure from the overinflated balloon being transmitted into the catheter's distal lumen. Overinflation of the balloon may cause PA rupture. Patients at highest risk of this are the elderly with pulmonary hypertension and weak, friable blood vessels.

In inspiration during spontaneous breathing, the PAP is lower than in expiration; it reaches the nearest value to alveolar/atmospheric pressure at end-expiration. Positive pressure mechanical ventilation reverses the normal physiological process and causes an increase in PAP during inspiration, but again the nearest value to alveolar/atmospheric pressure is at end-expiration. End-expiration provides the most accurate point in the respiratory cycle to give consistent and accurate measurements when wedging the PA catheter.

The mean intrathoracic pressure for patients who are ventilated and receiving positive end-expiratory pressure (PEEP) will be increased, artificially raising the PAP. For every 5 cm PEEP the PAP will be increased by approximately 1.5 mmHg. This can be significant for those patients receiving greater than 10 cm PEEP.

After wedging the PA catheter, the balloon should be slowly deflated and the monitored PA waveform should return to the screen (*Figure 17*).

PRACTICE POINT

Altering the patient's position from side to side, asking the patient to cough or breathe deeply, or giving a manual hyperinflation breath if ventilated may restore the characteristic PA waveform. If an antecubital approach has been taken, moving the arm to 90° to the body and flushing may assist in repositioning the catheter.

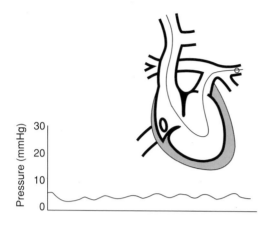

Figure 17. Progression of the PA catheter through the heart showing the changes in waveform that should be observed.

The proximal catheter tip should be kept near the lung hilum to reduce the risk of PA perforation. The position of the PA catheter must be checked daily on X-ray.

Troubleshooting

Migration of the catheter tip position is potentially harmful. Movement into a distal branch of the PA may occur within the first few hours of insertion as a result of body temperature softening the catheter. Spontaneous migration can also occur during cardiopulmonary bypass (CPB). Withdrawing the catheter by 4–5 cm prior to commencement of CPB may avoid this. The PA catheter can also migrate back into the RV, requiring readvancement into a PA position. This can only be achieved if the catheter has remained within its sterile plastic sheath.

PA catheter artefact (whip) can cause a distortion of up to 10 mmHg. Any increased contraction force (e.g. hyperdynamic heart) can cause the catheter to move and accelerate the fluid within. The greatest effect is on the PA systolic and diastolic pressures, therefore the mean PAP is more reliable. Additional causes of catheter artefact include:

- small air bubbles in transducer set,
- respiratory turbulence caused by mechanical ventilation,
- excessive stopcocks in the system,
- excessive lengths of tubing.

Other problems and checks are listed in *Table 9*.

Table 9. Problems encountered in wedging the PA catheter

Problem	Check for
No waveform	Correct connections to monitor
	Appropriate screen configuration selected
	Intact transducers
	Three-way taps within system turned on
Unable to wedge	Equipment failure
	Migration of catheter
	Ruptured balloon
Overwedging	Catheter against vessel wall – reposition and reinflate balloon with less air
Dampened waveform	Sufficient pressure in pressure bag
	Correct placement of transducer
	Check all connections
	Check position of PA catheter

3. CARDIAC OUTPUT MEASUREMENTS

3.1 Cardiac output

Cardiac output (CO) is the amount of blood (in litres) pumped out by the heart each minute, calculated from: $CO = SV \times HR$.

Normal CO = 4–8 l/min with potential to reach 25–30 l/min

A major determinant of CO is venous return (the amount of blood returned to the heart from the peripheral circulation). This can be adversely affected by intermittent positive ventilation. As a result of increased O_2 consumption/demand at cellular level CO can be increased. In the critically ill, sepsis is the main cause of a high CO. Additionally, high metabolic rates from thyrotoxicosis, fevers or phaeochromocytoma can also increase CO. A low CO is indicative of a reduced circulating volume or primary pump (cardiac) failure.

3.2 Cardiac index

The cardiac index (CI) is calculated by dividing the CO by the patient's body surface area (BSA): $CI = CO/BSA$.

Normal CI = 2.5–4.0 l/min/m^2

The CI reflects the precise amount of blood flow relative to a square metre of BSA. A measured CO can be the same value for a 35 kg or a 95 kg

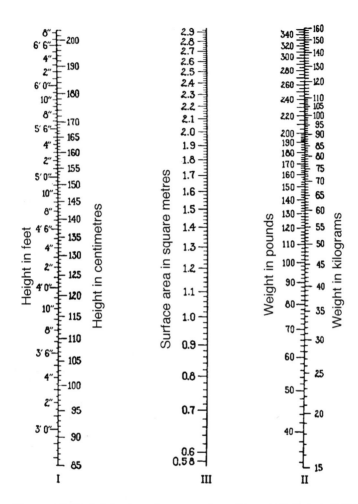

Figure 18. DuBois body surface area chart. (From E.F. Dubois (1936) *Basal Metabolism in Health and Disease.* Lea and Febiger, Philadelphia. Copyright 1920 by W.M. Boothby and R.B. Sandiford.)

patient, but the body surface area and tissue perfusion demands can vary. As BSA increases, so does the CO. The patient's BSA is calculated through a nomogram (e.g. DuBois BSA chart, *Figure 18*) using patient height (cm) and weight (kg). Computerized cardiac profiles will automatically calculate this once the patient's height and weight have been entered.

3.3 Methods of deriving cardiac output

The **Fick method**, based on Adolph Fick's work in the 1870s, states that O_2 consumption (per minute) equals the minute volume of O_2 extracted by the blood from the lungs. This method is most accurate only if the patient is physiologically stable. However, it is clinically impractical as all samples need to be drawn simultaneously.

CO is determined from:

$$CO = \frac{\text{oxygen consumption (ml/min)}}{\text{arterial–venous } O_2 \text{ difference}}$$

Arterial and venous O_2 content are measured to determine arterial and venous O_2 difference, and oxygen consumption is calculated using inspired and expired oxygen contents, and the ventilation rate.

The **dye indicator dilution method** is based on work in the 1890s by Stewart and modified by Hamilton. After injection of a dye or indicator into the system, continuous samples are taken to plot a 'time concentration' graph of indicator dilution. This method proves more accurate in high cardiac output states but is clinically impractical as it requires complex skills.

The **thermodilution method** was first described in the 1950s by Fegler and then further developed by Swan and Ganz. It applies the indicator dilution principles but uses temperature as the indicator. The injectate can be iced or at room temperature, although a temperature difference of 0.05°C can occur with an exaggerated respiration pattern. A known amount of solution is rapidly injected at a known temperature into the right atrium. This mixes with and cools the surrounding blood. The temperature is measured at a known distance downstream in the pulmonary artery by a thermistor bead embedded in the catheter. The resultant temperature change is plotted against time (*Figure 19*).

In a normal curve, temperature changes are represented by a sharp upstroke, caused by rapid injection of the injectate, followed by a prolonged fall back to the baseline (i.e. the curve demonstrates a change from body temperature to cooler temperature, and back to body temperature). The actual curve is in a negative direction but on most occasions is reproduced upright. The area under the curve is inversely proportional to the CO. When the CO is low, more time is required for the temperature to return to the baseline, producing a larger area under the curve. With high cardiac outputs the cooler injectate is carried faster through the heart and the temperature therefore returns to the baseline faster, producing a smaller area under the curve (*Figure 20*).

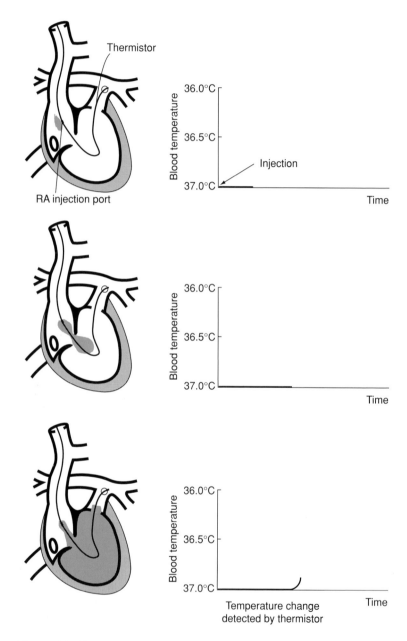

Figure 19. Using the thermodilution method to measure CO.

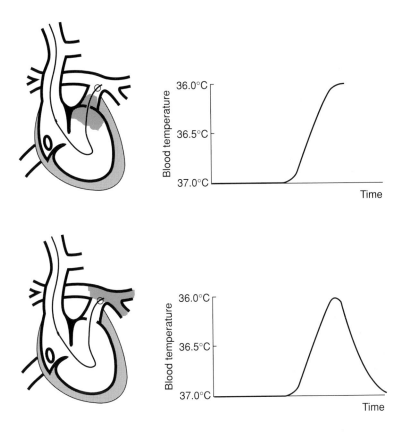

Figure 19. (*continued*).

An inaccurate curve features:

- abnormal artefacts,
- prolonged baseline drift due to recirculation,
- low amplitude due to small temperature difference.

A correction factor or constant is programmed into most CO systems and increases the reliability of CO readings, therefore eliminating the need for a second thermistor. Any changes in CO measuring technique (e.g. change in injectate volume) may require a new correction factor. Constants are supplied by most manufacturers with the PA catheter.

COVENTRY UNIVERSITY
NURSING & MIDWIFERY LIBRA

3.4 **Practical guide to measuring cardiac output**

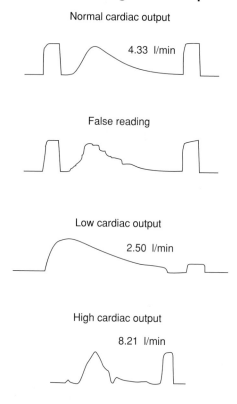

Figure 20. Characteristic CO waveforms.

The following basic checks should be undertaken prior to cardiac output studies.

- PA catheter position should be checked.
- Appropriate computation constant should be used for temperature and volume of fluid injected, catheter model and system used.
- Injectate probe cable should be connected by module to the monitor/computer.
- PA catheter should be connected via the thermistor lumen to the monitor/computer with an extension cable.
- Proximal injectate port should be checked for patency.
- Closed injectate delivery system (*Figure 21*) should be checked and the system flushed through with fluid of the desired temperature.

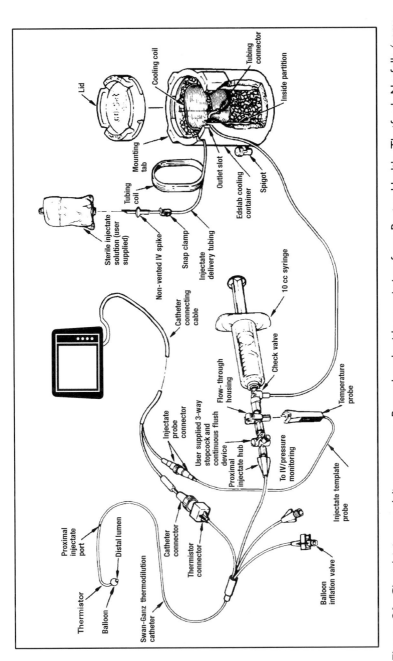

Figure 21. Closed injectate delivery system. Reproduced with permission from Baxter Health, Thetford, Norfolk (copyright 1988, Baxter Healthcare Corporation, Edwards Critical Care Division).

The following steps should be followed when undertaking CO studies.

- Select CO measurement function.
- Prepare the first 10 ml syringe; the syringe should only be handled by the wings.
- The system will indicate when it is ready to commence.
- Press the start switch and simultaneously inject within 4 sec the first of (usually) three successive measurements (used to determine the average).
- Each injection should be performed as quickly as possible to avoid temperature changes in the fluid.
- The computer will perform the calculations and indicate when the next recording can be made.
- Each recording should be obtained during the same phase of the respiratory cycle, preferably during end-expiration.
- If four readings are taken, the curves can be edited and those within a 10% variation should be chosen; these can then be used to obtain an average. The accuracy of the measurements can be determined by the shape of the curve.

Thermodilution techniques can be inaccurate in patients who have a backward flow of blood on the right side (e.g. tricuspid or pulmonary valve regurgitation, ventricular/atrial septal defects). Inaccurate measurements can also occur if a jugular approach is taken with extracorporeal membrane oxygenation due to insufficient mixing of natural venous return and membrane oxygenator return; if a femoral approach has been taken, CO is accurate.

The use of left ventricular assist devices does not cause problems in CO determination, but right ventricular assist devices (RVADs) render CO measurements invalid by this technique. The injectate moves from the RA into the pump before moving back into the PA. In patients with RVADs *in situ*, CO determination through the Fick principle is likely to be most accurate.

4. DERIVED MEASUREMENTS

4.1 Systemic vascular resistance (SVR) and SVR index (SVRI)

Normal SVR $= 900-1600$ dynes/sec/cm^5
Normal SVRI $= 2000-2400$ dynes/sec/cm^5/m^2

Resistance is the relationship of pressure to flow, as determined with reference to Ohm's law. This value is a representation of **afterload**, the amount of resistance the left ventricle must overcome to eject blood into the aorta.

$$\text{Resistance} = \frac{\text{mean pressure across the vascular bed}}{\text{blood flow}}$$

Since resistance relates pressure to flow, pressure is calculated by measuring the gradient between the proximal (mean arterial) and distal (central venous) ends of the cardiovascular system. It is then divided by CO to take account of blood flow. SVR reflects an average of all the vascular beds; regional differences are not reflected in this.

$$\text{SVR} = \frac{(\text{MAP} - \text{RAP}) \times 79.96}{\text{CO}}$$

The unit of resistance is dynes/sec/cm^5. To convert mmHg and l/min into units of resistance, the value is multiplied by a conversion factor of 79.96. This factor can be indexed relative to the patient's BSA.

$$\text{SVRI} = \frac{\text{SVR}}{\text{BSA}}$$

A decreasing SVR suggests a general vasodilatory reaction (e.g. sepsis and endotoxin release). Over-administration of vasodilator drugs (e.g. glyceryl trinitrate, sodium nitroprusside) or hyperthermia with vasodilation may also reduce SVR. An increasing SVR is indicative of general vasoconstriction, for example in response to cardiogenic and hypovolaemic shock.

4.2 Pulmonary vascular resistance (PVR) and PVR index (PVRI)

Normal PVR = 20–120 dynes/sec/cm^5
Normal PVRI = 225–315 dynes/sec/cm^5

Pulmonary vascular resistance (PVR) reflects the resistance to blood flow in the pulmonary circulation. In healthy patients, the pulmonary circulation is usually more compliant than the systemic circulation and so values are considerably lower. The resistance offered by the pulmonary bed is usually one-sixth of that offered by the systemic bed.

The same principles are used to calculate PVR as SVR, where the mean PAP is seen as the proximal end and the PAWP is seen as the distal end of the pulmonary vasculature.

$$\text{PVR} = \frac{(\text{mean PAP} - \text{PAWP}) \times 79.96}{\text{CO}}$$

This factor can be indexed relative to the patient's BSA.

$$\text{PVRI} = \frac{\text{PVR}}{\text{BSA}}$$

Factors increasing the PVR include pulmonary embolism, pulmonary hypertension, pulmonary oedema and leaky pulmonary capillary syndrome in sepsis where alveolar hypoxia causes vasoconstriction of the precapillary pulmonary arterioles. Reduced pulmonary pressures are often seen in hypo-volaemic patients or those receiving vasodilatory therapies.

4.3 Stroke volume (SV), stroke volume index (SVI) and derivatives

These values are not directly measured but are derived from the previous parameters.

Normal SV = 60–100 ml/beat
Normal SVI = 35–70 ml/beat/m²

Stroke volume is the amount of blood pumped by the ventricle in one contraction. It indicates the contractility state of the heart and is related to myocardial fibre function and ventricular size. During diastole the ventricles fill to 120–130 ml (ventricular end-diastolic volume). During systole, 70–80 ml of blood is ejected, accounting for a normal 60% **ejection fraction**.

SV is calculated by:

$$SV = \frac{CO}{HR} \times 100 \text{ ml/l}$$

SV is influenced by **preload, afterload** and **contractility**, and can there-fore be affected by factors influencing blood volume and central venous return, tachycardia and arrhythmias.

Decreased myocardial contractility is associated with hypoxia, hypercapnia and acidosis. An increased SV is associated with bradycardia and the effec-tive administration of positive inotropic agents.

Left cardiac work index (LCWI)

Normal LCWI = 3.4–4.2 kg/m/m²

This assesses the amount of work the left ventricle performs each minute when ejecting blood. It is calculated by: work = pressure generated × volume of blood pumped/min, divided by BSA in order to index it:

$$LCWI = \frac{MAP \times CO \times 0.0136}{BSA}$$

To convert pressure (l/mmHg) to work (kg/m), a value is multiplied by a conversion factor of 0.0136.

Abnormal LCWI values reflect changes in pressure and/or volume.

Left ventricular stroke work index (LVSWI)

Normal LVSWI = 50–62 g/m/m^2

This value reflects the amount of work the left ventricle undertakes with each beat (i.e. per SV). It is calculated using the same formula as for LCWI but using mean arterial pressure and SV: work = pressure generated × volume of blood pumped/beat, indexed by dividing by BSA:

$$LVSWI = \frac{MAP \times SV \times 0.0136}{BSA}$$

Use of the constant 0.0136 is again required.

LVSWI assesses left ventricular contractility and reflects abnormal volume and contractility states. It indicates which treatments may need to be given (e.g. inotropes or volume loading). Increased LVSWI may also indicate increased oxygen consumption associated with angina.

Right cardiac work index (RCWI)

Normal RCWI = 0.54–0.66 kg/m/m^2

This assesses the work that the RV performs each minute when ejecting blood. The same principles are used as for LCWI: RCWI = pressure generated × volume of blood, divided by BSA to index it. Using corresponding right-side figures this translates to:

$$RCWI = \frac{MPAP \times CO \times 0.0136}{BSA}$$

An abnormal value reflects alterations in either pressure or volume.

Right ventricular stroke work index (RVSWI)

Normal RVSWI = 7.9–9.7 g/m/m^2

This assesses the amount of work the RV performs per beat, when ejecting blood. The same principles are used as for LVSWI but right-sided values are used:

$$RVSWI = \frac{MPAP \times SV \times 0.0136}{BSA}$$

Changes in this variable reflect alterations in the pressure, preload, afterload or contractility state.

5. MIXED VENOUS OXYGEN SATURATION (SvO_2)

Normal SvO_2 = 60–80%

CO provides information regarding the adequacy of oxygen delivery to the tissues, but gives no information regarding the degree of oxygen uptake at cellular level. Assessment of tissue metabolism is determined by mixed venous oxygen saturation. This facility has been available since the early 1980s.

Measurement of oxygen saturation of the blood is used to give a global assessment of tissue oxygenation. When oxygen delivery to the tissues and oxygen extraction from the cells is normal, the oxygen saturation of blood returning to the heart will be 75%. Local variations exist, for example venous blood returning from the kidneys has a higher concentration of oxygen (91%) than venous blood returning from the heart (30%). Complete venous mixing occurs in the RV and therefore sampling of blood from the PA is considered to give an accurate estimation of true SvO_2.

Cardiac surgical patients, patients with post-myocardial infarction complications (e.g. cardiogenic shock), those receiving vasoactive drugs or with respiratory failure requiring optimal PEEP levels, can all benefit from SvO_2 monitoring.

Measurements can be undertaken on an intermittent basis (via sampling from the PA port) or on a continuous basis using an SvO_2 catheter. This is a modified 7.5 or 8 FG catheter with optic fibres that transmit light to and from the blood stream. The light from the catheter is absorbed by haemoglobin. A second optical fibre transmits that light which is not absorbed to a light detector and data processor for analysis. The ratio of haemoglobin to oxyhaemoglobin can be calculated because of the light absorption characteristics. This provides real-time information on changes in SvO_2.

Most systems have facilities for complete automatic calibration of the system prior to insertion, to ensure catheter measurement accuracy, together with precalibration checks of the bedside computer to ensure accuracy of the continuous display of SvO_2.

A decrease in any of the determinants of oxygen supply – CO, haemoglobin (Hb) or arterial oxygen saturation (SaO_2) – is usually associated with a decrease in SvO_2. SvO_2 levels below 60% occur due to increased oxygen extraction by the tissues and reflect O_2 supply/demand imbalance. When the SvO_2 remains below 50%, lactic acidosis can occur as a result of anaerobic metabolism. Permanent cellular damage occurs at levels under 20%.

A gradual increase in SvO_2 beyond 80% can indicate decreased peripheral oxygen consumption, for example in hypothermia, or increased peripheral shunting due to impaired cell utilization of oxygen, as seen in septic shock and cyanide toxicity.

> **PRACTICE POINT**
> Reductions in SvO_2 of 10% or greater for more than 5 min require prompt assessment of the patient and in particular of the three determinants of oxygen delivery.

5.1 Troubleshooting with SvO_2 monitoring

The following precautions should be taken.

- Any calibration of the SvO_2 catheter should be performed before insertion, following the manufacturer's instructions.
- The catheter should be accurately placed: if inserted too distally then placement shines light on the vessel wall and not on the red blood cells.
- Any condition which may interrupt light transmission (e.g. catheter kinking, clot formation) should be prevented.
- Light intensity signals should be monitored: a low alarm can indicate a bent, broken or occluded catheter, a high/distal placement or low flow through the PA.

5.2 Interpreting SvO_2 changes

Changes in SvO_2 are interpreted as shown in *Table 10*.

SvO_2 in patients receiving venovenous extracorporeal membrane oxygenation is not strictly mixed venous oxygen, as this will include a contribution from the membrane oxygenator. Analysis of the SvO_2 will reveal a mixture of venous and highly saturated oxygen-rich blood from ECMO. This figure cannot be used to reflect oxygen delivery, but can be used to reflect trends. Examples of SvO_2 recordings are shown in *Figure 22*.

> **PRACTICE POINT**
> Proactive care is imperative. All patient activities must be planned in line with the patient's tolerance and reserve.

Table 10. Changes in SvO$_2$

SvO$_2$ (%)	Patient problem	Patient activity	Rationale
Increasing (> 80%)	Sepsis	Muscle paralysis	Decreased O$_2$ consumption
	Vasodilated states	Anaesthesia	Increased O$_2$ delivery
	Cyanide toxicity	Effective ventilation	Increased Hb
	Increased PaO$_2$/SaO$_2$	Blood transfusion	
Normal (60–80%)	Adequate oxygenation		O$_2$ supply = O$_2$ demand
	Adequate perfusion		
Decreasing (< 60%)	Hyperthermia	Increased sedation	Increased O$_2$ consumption
	Seizures	Increased respiratory work	Increased CO
	Low CO	Patient movement	Decreased O$_2$ delivery
	Hypoxaemia	Pain/anxiey	Decreased CO
		PEEP	Decreased SaO$_2$
		Haemorrhage	Decreased Hb
		Patient suctioning	

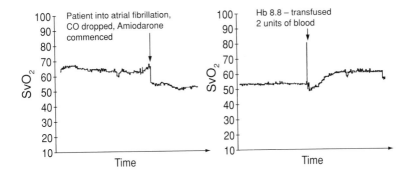

Figure 22. SvO$_2$ recordings: critical patient events.

6. FURTHER READING

Boutros, A.R. and Lee, C. (1986) Values of continuous mixed venous oxygen in the management of critically ill patients. *Critical Care Medicine*, **14**, 132–134.

Bryant, A. and Kennedy, G.T. (1981) The effect of body position upon pulmonary artery pressure and pulmonary capillary wedge pressure measurements. *Circulation* (Part II), **66**, II-97.

Cengiz, M., Crapo, P. and Gardner, R. (1983) The effect of ventilation on the accuracy of pulmonary artery and wedge pressure measurements. *Critical Care Medicine*, **1**, 502–507.

Chulay, M. and Miller, T. (1984) The effect of back rest elevation on pulmonary artery and pulmonary capillary wedge in patients after cardiac surgery. *Heart Lung*, **13**, 138–140.

Davidson, L.J. and Brown, S. (1986) Continous SvO$_2$ monitoring: a tool for analysing haemodynamic status. *Heart Lung*, **15**, 287–292.

Dorinsky, P.M. (1983) The effect of positive end expiratory pressure on cardiac output. *Chest*, **84**, 21–26.

Edwards, J.D., Shoemaker, W.C. and Vincent, J.L. (1993) *Oxygen Transport: Principles and Practice*. W.B. Saunders, Philadelphia.

Fick, A. (1870) Uber die messung des blutquantums in den Heerzventrikein. Reprinted and translated in Hoff, H.E. and Scott, H.J. (1948) Physiology. *New England Journal of Medicine*, **24**, 120.

Gershan. J.A. (1983) The effect of positive end expiratory pressure on pulmonary capillary wedge pressure. *Heart Lung*, **12**, 143–148.

Jaquith, S.M. (1985) Continous measurement of mixed venous oxygen. Clinical application and advances for critical care nursing. *Critical Care Nurse*, **5**, 40–44.

Kennedy, G.T., Bryant, A. and Crawford, M. (1984) The effects of lateral body positioning on measurements of pulmonary artery and pulmonary artery wedge pressures. *Heart Lung,* **13**, 155–158.

Pearl, R.G., Rosenthal, M.H. and Nielson, L. (1986) Effect of injectate volume and temperature on thermodilution cardiac output determination. *Anaesthesiology*, **64**, 798–801.

Synder, J.V. (1982) Effects of mechanical ventilation on the measurement of cardiac output by thermodilution. *Critical Care Medicine*, **10**, 677–682.

CHAPTER 4

Patient Case Studies

I. HYPOVOLAEMIC SHOCK

I.I Practical presentation

Mrs E was a 64-year-old lady involved in a high-speed road traffic accident. Initially, she required fluid resuscitation at the scene of the accident and later full skeletal examination revealed a fractured right clavicle, fractured ribs 3 and 4 on the right side, a fractured right femur and a suspected liver tear. At the scene of the accident she had a Glasgow coma scale of 12.

Once stabilized, she was taken to theatre for repair of the suspected liver laceration and internal fixation of her femur. Following surgery she was admitted to the intensive care unit (ICU) for post-operative fluid management and monitoring. At this stage, she had been transfused seven units of whole blood, and 1.5 l of crystalloid fluids. Her systemic pressures and urine output remained low and a PA catheter was inserted. Her PaO_2 was 12.5 kPa self-ventilating with an FiO_2 of 0.45.

Haemodynamic profile

BP	91/72 mmHg	Decreased
MAP	77 mmHg	Decreased
HR	115/min	Increased
RAP/CVP	2 mmHg	Decreased
CO	2.8 l/min	Decreased
CI	1.6 l/min/m²	Decreased
SV	28 ml/beat	Decreased
SVR	1853 dynes/sec/cm⁵	Increased
PAP	18/4 mmHg	Decreased
PAWP	3 mmHg	Decreased
PVR	196 dynes/sec/cm⁵	Decreased
LVSWI	42.4 g/m/m²	Decreased
RVSWI	4.6 g/m/m²	Decreased
LCWI	2.9 g/m/m²	Decreased
RCWI	0.31 g/m/m²	Decreased
SvO_2	55	Decreased

Treatment

Based on information from the haemodynamic profile Mrs E was given incremental fluid challenges of 250 ml to a total of 1.5 l (two units of blood to bring her Hb to 10.5 g/l) followed by a synthetic colloid for the remainder. No obvious signs of further blood loss were noted and her condition slowly improved.

Restoring her circulating volume had the effect of increasing her SV, intracardiac pressures, CO and BP. Consequently her SVR was reduced as this compensatory mechanism was no longer required. Her SvO_2 increased as greater perfusion to the peripheries led to a reduction in oxygen extraction and therefore an increase in the amount of oxygen returning to the heart.

> **PRACTICE POINT**
> If a patient with cardiac history is admitted and needs aggressive fluid resuscitation, monitor PAWP and RAP for failure. Give fluid challenges, cautiously monitoring filling pressures, auscultating lungs for crackles and S3 heart sounds (abnormal third heart sound – loss of ventricular compliance as in cardiac failure).

1.2 Theoretical application

Mrs E presented with hypovolaemic shock. This is a reduction in circulating intravascular volume caused through blood loss or loss of fluid into the third space (*Table 11*).

Table 11. Causes of hypovolaemic shock

Blood loss	Third space loss	Fluid loss
Haemorrhage	Intestinal obstruction	Vomiting
Gut bleed	Burns	Diabetes
Haemothorax	Ascites	Excessive sweating
Fracture site	Sepsis	Diarrhoea
Retroperitoneal		

Clinical presentation

The patient's condition was primarily due to reduced circulating volume and secondarily due to the sympathetic nervous system compensatory mechanisms. Symptoms and signs to note are:

- small pulse volume,
- fast heart rate,
- poor capillary refill,
- skin turgor dry,
- anxiety,
- pale, cool, clammy appearance,
- tachypnoeic,
- decreased urine output,
- may complain of thirst,
- base deficit below −5.

pH may be normal if respiratory compensation is successful.

Haemodynamic profile – interpretation

BP/MAP	Decreased relative to patient's normal. Pulse pressure narrowed. Slow rise and dampened arterial waveform.
HR	Increased as a compensatory mechanism.
RAP	Decreased due to low circulating volume and preload.
CO/CI	Decreased due to reduced ventricular filling.
SVR	Increased as a compensatory mechanism.
PAP	Decreased: waveform may show similar dampening and slow upstroke as arterial line.
PAWP	Decreased due to reduced circulating volume.
PVR	Unaltered until hypoxaemia/acidaemia occur, then PVR will increase due to vasoconstrictor effect.
L(R)VSWI/ L(R)CWI	Decreased due to low circulating volume. Related to low SV, CO and PAWP.
SvO$_2$	Decreased levels due to capillary hypoperfusion and therefore increased oxygen extraction.

Treatment options

The aims of the treatment include:

- Ensure adequate ventilation and oxygenation to meet the patient's needs.
- Check or reduce volume loss.
- Administer appropriate fluids – see Appendix A.

PRACTICE POINT

Use frequent checks of Hb and haematocrit to guide appropriate fluid for replacement and to avoid problems associated with increased viscosity.

---

2. CARDIOGENIC SHOCK

2.1 Practical presentation

Mrs P was a 62-year-old lady with a three-year history of increasing chest pain. She was on calcium channel blockers while awaiting cardiac surgery.

She was admitted into the coronary care unit following an episode of severe radiating chest pain. Electrocardiogram in the accident and emergency (A&E) department revealed evolving Q waves in V4–6, lead I and AVL. There were ST segment changes and initially T wave elevation in those leads. A diagnosis of acute antero-lateral myocardial infarction was made and the appropriate treatment commenced.

Twenty-four hours following admission, Mrs P's condition deteriorated with a falling blood pressure, reduced urine output and increased tachypnoea. Mrs P was frightened and anxious, and was complaining of becoming more breathless. She was also starting to become sweaty, and cool peripherally. On auscultation, crackles were heard in both lung bases with a poor response to intravenous frusemide. Mrs P was commenced on a dobutamine infusion via a peripheral line. Her CVP reading remained at 18 mmHg.

The patient's condition deteriorated. A pulmonary artery catheter was floated to obtain a more accurate assessment of cardiac function.

Haemodynamic profile

BP	87/73 mmHg	Decreased
MAP	77 mmHg	Decreased
HR	124/min	Increased
RAP/CVP	18 mmHg	Increased
CO	3 l/min	Decreased
CI	1.8 l/min/m^2	Decreased
SV	25 ml/beat	Decreased
SVR	1800 dynes/sec/cm^5	Increased
PAP	38/15 mmHg	Increased
PAWP	21 mmHg	Increased
PVR	228 dynes/sec/cm^5	Increased
LVSWI	31.7 g/m/m^2	Decreased
RVSWI	12.4 g/m/m^2	Increased
LCWI	2.7 g/m/m^2	Decreased
RCWI	0.81 g/m/m^2	Increased
SvO$_2$	56	Decreased

Mrs P's arterial blood gases taken whilst breathing an FiO$_2$ of 0.4 showed hypoxia (PO$_2$ 8 kPa) and metabolic acidosis (pH 7.3, PCO$_2$ 4.5 kPa, bicarbonate 19, base deficit −11).

Treatment

With Mrs P's past history, deteriorating condition and raised and increased filling pressures with low CO/CI, the problem was diagnosed as one of cardiac failure related to cardiogenic shock. Both preload and afterload needed to be reduced and contractility strengthened.

Following this profile, the dobutamine was increased to 7.5 μg/kg/min to increase contractility. Dopamine was also added in at a renal dose of 2.5 μg/kg/min to help improve renal perfusion. Following these measures some improvement was noted in CO/CI, but the SVR (a measure of afterload) remained high. Therefore, a nitroglycerine infusion was commenced at 1 μg/kg/min and titrated until the SVR decreased and a further increase in CO/CI was seen. Mrs P's condition stabilized over the next 12 h, when weaning of the inotropic therapy could begin and oral anti-cardiac failure treatment could be introduced until she underwent cardiac surgery for coronary artery grafting.

PRACTICE POINTS
- Patients with a long-standing cardiac history may need higher filling pressures to maintain their CO/CI.
- The myocardium is inevitably irritable following myocardial infarction; maintaining the serum potassium at the upper end of normal (4–4.5 mmol/l) will reduce the risk of dysrhythmias which can further decrease SV and CO/CI.
- Cardiogenic shock has a high mortality rate (80%), therefore care needs to be proactive.
- Physical activity needs to be planned carefully into the patient's day – even simple acts can increase myocardial oxygen consumption.

2.2 Theoretical application

Pump failure, with a decreased CO insufficient to meet the body's metabolic needs, is caused through:

- acute myocardial infarction, when at least 40% of the myocardium is injured,
- severe dysrhythmias – tachyarrhythmias/bradyarrhythmias,
- end-stage cardiomyopathy,
- valvular disease (e.g. aortic regurgitation causing the LV to fail),
- mechanical defects – acquired ventricular septal defect,
- cardiac tamponade.

Clinical presentation

Cardiogenic shock is primarily due to pump failure and secondarily due to sympathetic nervous system compensatory mechanisms. The patient may present a picture of left- and right-sided failure incorporating pulmonary symptoms and signs such as:

- small pulse volume,
- fast HR,
- poor capillary refill,
- pale, cool, clammy,
- metabolic acidosis,

- anxiety, apprehension,
- tachypnoeic, shallow breathing,
- neck veins visibly distended,
- decreased urine output,
- hypoxaemia,
- base deficit below −5,
- restlessness, confusion.

Haemodynamic profile – interpretation

BP/MAP	Decreased relative to patient's norm. Pulse pressure narrowed. Slow rise and dampened arterial waveform.
HR	Increased as a compensatory mechanism.
RAP	Unaltered if LV failure, increased in RV failure.
CO/CI	Decreased due to reduced isovolumetric and ejection phase of systole with decreased SV.
SVR	Increased as a compensatory mechanism.
PAP	Increased due to back pressure from LV failure.
PAWP	Increased due to back pressure from LV failure.
PVR	Unaltered if isolated problem, but eventually hypoxaemia/acidaemia will cause an increase.
LVSWI/LCWI	Decreased due to poor generation of pressures, related to low SV and CO/CI.
RVSWI/RCWI	Increased due to pulmonary vasoconstriction and back pressure from LV failure.
SvO_2	Decreased due to capillary hypoperfusion and increased oxygen extraction. Pulmonary oedema will further reduce SvO_2.

Treatment options

To improve myocardial oxygen supply:

- ensure optimum arterial oxygenation.

To decrease myocardial oxygen demand:

- relieve pain and anxiety,
- provide rest by effectively managing care,
- control dysrhythmias and maintain serum potassium at high–normal levels.

To increase CO and peripheral perfusion:

- optimize preload with volume or diuretics,
- maximize contractility with inotropes,
- reduce afterload with vasodilators, intra-aortic balloon pump.

Table 12. Other specific cardiac problems

Patient problem	Cardiac output studies – specific pointers	Cause
Right ventricular infarction (occlusion of coronary artery, usually RCA)	Decreased PAP, PAWP Decreased SV, CO/CI	RV failure Septal shifting into LV space
PRACTICE POINT Treatment is usually focused on supporting left cardiac function by volume loading and intropes. Cautiously reducing right ventricular afterload with vasodilators may support the RV function.		
Acquired ventricular septal defect (VSD)	Increased PAP, PAWP Inaccurate CO/CI (thermodilution)	Movement of blood in LV into RV Recirculation of blood via pulmonary circulation to LV to RV
PRACTICE POINT The size of the left to right shunt is dependent on the SVR:PVR ratio. An increased SVR will limit forward flow and increase the shunt across the defect.		
Aortic valve dysfunction	Increased SVR	Compensatory mechanism to maintain MAP
PRACTICE POINT Caring for a patient with aortic stenosis requires fine manipulation of preload and afterload to maintain an acceptable CO. Filling pressures must be maintained to fill the hypertrophied left ventricle.		

Table 12. (continued)

Mitral valve dysfunction/papillary muscle rupture	Increased PAWP	Needed to maintain LV preload and CO/CI

PRACTICE POINT

A left atrial line may be used to measure left atrial pressures (LAP). This is threaded through one of the pulmonary veins or inserted directly into the left atrium. No air must be injected into and no drugs should be administered through this line and removal should be at the earliest time appropriate to the patient's condition.

Cardiac tamponade	Pulsus paradoxus	Reduction of > 10 mmHg systolic BP during inspiration due to accumulation of fluid in pericardial sac equalizing all intracardiac pressure.
• Acute post-surgery trauma	Similar RAP, PADP, LAP	
• Chronic infection, neoplastic		

PRACTICE POINT

The amount of fluid required to cause cardiac impairment is related more to speed of accumulation than to volume. Surgical drainage will relieve the tamponade.

PRACTICE POINTS
- Use touch and sight in assessment to indicate patient changes.
- Be observant and proactive in care.

2.3 Other specific cardiac problems

Other specific cardiac problems are listed in *Table 12*.

3. SEPTIC SHOCK – SEPTIC INFLAMMATORY RESPONSE SYNDROME (SIRS)

3.1 Practical presentation

Mrs M was a 37-year-old lady with an 18 month history of Crohn's disease. She had undergone an extensive bowel resection and formation of ileostomy 72 h previously. Following an uneventful initial recovery period, she became increasingly unwell on the ward. After assessment on the ward by the ICU team, she was admitted to the ICU for management.

On admission, her respiratory function was poor, with arterial blood gases showing hypoxaemia and a marked metabolic acidosis, despite receiving 100% oxygen via a face mask. Her BP was 85/65 despite fluid challenges and a CVP measurement of 10 mmHg. She was unresponsive to commands and became increasingly disoriented. Her core temperature was 38.7°C and specimens for microbiological cultures had already been taken. She was receiving dobutamine at 5 μg/kg/min and her Hb was 11.7 g/dl.

She was immediately intubated and ventilated with an FiO_2 of 0.8 and 4 cm of PEEP and invasive monitoring lines were inserted; a PA catheter was inserted to provide more detailed assessment to guide treatment.

Haemodynamic profile

BP	97/63 mmHg	Normal
MAP	74 mmHg	Normal
HR	131/min	Increased
RAP/CVP	10 mmHg	Normal
CO	12.5 l/min	Increased
CI	6.0 l/min/m^2	Increased
SV	95.4 ml/beat	Normal
SVR	410 dynes/sec/cm^5	Decreased
PAP	32/23 mmHg	Increased
PAWP	11 mmHg	Normal
PVR	102 dynes/sec/cm^5	Normal
LVSWI	59.1 g/m/m^2	Normal

RVSWI	10.8 g/m/m²	Normal
LCWI	6.7 g/m/m²	Increased
RCWI	0.71 g/m/m²	Increased
SvO₂	85	Increased

Treatment

The haemodynamic profile indicated that Mrs M had a high output state. Her cardiovascular state was stable with ventilation and oxygen support, fluids and inotropes. Dopamine at 2.5 µg/kg/min was commenced to support renal function. Her SVR remained low and the CO/CI was maintained through an increased HR. Increasing the SVR with a vasoconstrictor would possibly reduce the compensatory mechanisms and, by effectively increasing the afterload, reduce the need for over-aggressive volume infusion. Noradrenaline was commenced at 0.05 µg/kg/min and increased to 0.12 µg/kg/min with a rise in SVR to 1204. Her HR dropped to 98/min and the dobutamine was gradually weaned. After a further 6 days of cardiovascular and respiratory support, her condition stabilized, requiring no inotropic support, and Mrs M was discharged to the ward.

PRACTICE POINT

Critically ill patients do not tolerate sudden discontinuation of inotropes – wean slowly as tolerated and ensure a prepared syringe is set up, and prepare to 'piggy-back' the system.

3.2 Theoretical application

Septic shock/SIRS was initially defined as any shocked state associated with an infection, although patients may present with classic septic shock symptoms with no micro-organism cultured. Gram-negative organisms are the most common cause of sepsis (*Escherichia coli*, *Pseudomonas aeruginosa*, *Klebsiella* spp).

Patients at particular risk include those with:

- inadequate immune response (diabetes, liver or renal disease, the elderly, post trauma),
- primary infections (pneumonia, urinary tract infection, peritonitis, abscess formation),
- iatrogenic sources (in-dwelling vascular/urinary catheters, extensive major abdominal or pelvic surgery).

The cascade of host inflammatory responses post-insult characterize the systemic problems associated with sepsis.

Clinical presentation – hyperdynamic phase
Septic shock/SIRS is related to cardiac dysfunction, peripheral vascular failure and the resultant hypovolaemia. Symptoms and signs include:

- bounding pulse,
- fast HR,
- warm to touch with flushed appearance,
- tachypnoeic with hyperventilation,
- decreased urine output,
- may be alkalosis from hyperventilation or metabolic acidosis if sepsis and tissue hypoxia well established,
- confusion, restlessness, delirium.

Haemodynamic profile – interpretation

BP/MAP	Normal/slightly decreased dependent on intravascular volume replacement. Pulse pressure may be widened. Low diastolic.
HR	Increased as a compensatory mechanism.
RAP	Normal/decreased dependent on volume status.
CO/CI	Increased to maintain BP against falling SVR.
SVR	Decreased due to biochemical mediator-induced vasodilatation.
PAP	Normal/decreased dependent on volume status.
PAWP	Normal/decreased dependent on volume status.
PVR	Unaltered but increases with hypoxaemia/acidaemia.
LVSWI/ RVSWI	Normal/decreased if volume status low with poor generation of pressures.
LCWI/ RCWI	Increased due to CO/CI.
SvO_2	Increased due to cellular response interfering with oxygen uptake and utilization.

Treatment options

- Ensure adequate oxygenation and ventilation.
- Ensure all sites cultured and discussion with microbiologist directs antimicrobial treatment and removal of any identified septic focus.
- Increase SVR through use of noradrenaline infusion to produce vasoconstriction.
- Administer adequate fluid replacement to restore filling pressures.
- Monitor and treat for other system involvement – renal failure, cardiac failure, disseminated intravascular clotting, adult respiratory distress syndrome.

4. ADULT RESPIRATORY DISTRESS SYNDROME (ARDS) OR ACUTE LUNG INJURY (ALI)

4.1 Practical presentation

Mr J, a 17-year-old student, presented in the A&E department with atypical pneumonia. Despite increasing inspired oxygen concentrations to 80%, he became confused and restless on the ward. Blood gas analysis showed continued hypoxaemia (PaO_2 6.8, SaO_2 89%) and increasing respiratory distress. Chest X-ray showed patchy bilateral infiltrates. He was referred to ICU for respiratory care.

On admission, he was intubated and ventilated on 100% O_2 and 5 cm H_2O PEEP. To guide the treatment plan, a PA catheter was inserted.

Haemodynamic profile

BP	115/50 mmHg	Normal
MAP	74 mmHg	Normal
HR	120/min	Increased
RAP/CVP	17 mmHg	Increased
CO	8.4 l/min	Increased
CI	3.8 l/min/m²	Normal
SV	70 ml/beat	Normal
SVR	750 dynes/sec/cm⁵	Decreased
PAP	34/21 mmHg	Increased
PAWP	10 mmHg	Normal
PVR	259 dynes/sec/cm⁵	Increased
LVSWI	60 g/m/m²	Normal
RVSWI	10.1 g/m/m²	Increased
LCWI	4.2 g/m/m²	Normal
RCWI	0.72 g/m/m²	Increased
SvO_2	55	Decreased

Treatment

After several days of ventilation requiring high FiO_2, Mr J's respiratory status stabilized. At times he became hypoxic and required increased oxygen levels prior to any procedure. Following sputum culture and sensitivity, appropriate antibiotics were commenced, and with appropriate fluid management and oxygenation, no left-sided failure developed. After 7 days' treatment with antibiotics and intensive physiotherapy as tolerated, resolution of the ARDS occurred and within a further 3 days he was able to be weaned from the ventilator and extubated.

4.2 Theoretical application

ARDS is a complex, poorly understood syndrome which is also known as shock lung, high-permeability pulmonary oedema and post-perfusion lung. It usually occurs between 24 hours and 7 days after the initial insult, and risk factors include:

- post trauma,
- inhalation of substances (gastric contents, near-drowning),
- infection (septicaemia),
- haematological (massive blood transfusion, disseminated intravascular coagulopathy),
- metabolic (pancreatitis).

ARDS is characterized by disruption of the alveolar capillary membrane leading to fluid accumulation, protein leakage and microthrombi causing:

- atelectasis,
- reduced functional residual capacity,
- impaired gas exchange,
- increased shunt through ventilation/perfusion mismatch,
- gross hypoxaemia.

Clinical presentation
The presenting symptoms are related to the loss of lung compliance.

Respiratory assessment will show:

- dyspnoea with crackles and wheezes on auscultation,
- use of accessory muscles if self-ventilating,
- hypoxaemia, hypocapnia, respiratory alkalosis,
- chest X-ray with scattered infiltrates – 'ground glass' appearance.

Haemodynamic profile – interpretation

BP/MAP	Unaltered if no LV dysfunction.
HR	Unaltered if no LV dysfunction.
RAP	Unaltered if no LV dysfunction.
CO/CI	Unaltered but decreases due to decreased LV filling volume secondary to increased PVR.
SVR	Unaltered if no LV dysfunction/sepsis.
PAP	Increased in the prescence of high PVR.
PAWP	Unaltered if no LV dysfunction.
PVR	Increased due to hypoxaemia.
RVSWI/RCWI	Increased due to high right-sided pressures.
LVSWI/LCWI	Unaltered if no LV dysfunction.
SvO_2	Decreased due to hypoxia and increased cellular oxygen extraction.

Table 13. Other specific respiratory problems

Patient problem	Cardiac output studies – specific pointers	Cause
Pulmonary embolism – massive occlusion of main branch of PA	Increased PAP	Required to maintain flow through pulmonary bed
	Increased PVR, PAP, RVSWI	Inadequate left-sided filling and oxygenation
	• Decreased BP, CO/CI and PAWP	Compensatory mechanism
	• Decreased SV, LVSWI and SvO_2	
	Increased SVR	

> **PRACTICE POINT**
> Due to increased respiratory effort, accurate measurement of PAWP may be difficult. In this situation, interpretation of trends is of more use.

Chronic obstructive airways disease – chronic bronchitis, emphysema and asthma	Increased PAP, PVR and RVSWI	RV hypertrophy, hypoxaemia and pulmonary vasoconstriction
	Decreased SvO_2	Hypoxaemia

PRACTICE POINT

Desaturation on patient turning: is preoxygenation required? Is recovery taking longer? Does the patient hold saturations better on one side? Build this into care planning and evaluation.

Treatment options

- Optimal ventilation and oxygenation.
- Use of PEEP.
- Optimal fluid therapy (see Appendix A).
- Use of patient positioning (e.g. prone) to minimize shunting.

4.3 Other specific respiratory problems

Other specific respiratory problems are listed in *Table 13*.

5. FURTHER READING

Carlson, R.W. and Gehab, M.A. (eds) (1993) *Principles and Practice of Medical Intensive Care.* W.B. Saunders, Philadelphia.

Civetta, J.M., Taylor, R.W. and Kirby, R.R. (eds) (1992) *Critical Care,* 2nd Edn. J.B. Lippincott, Philadelphia.

Dennison, R.D. (1994) Making sense of haemodynamic monitoring. *American Journal of Nursing,* **94**, 24–31.

Dantzker, D.R. (ed.) (1991) *Cardiopulmonary Critical Care,* 2nd Edn. W.B. Saunders, Philadelphia.

Forreter, J. S., Diamond, G. and McHugh, T.J. (1971) Filling pressures in the right and left sides of the heart in acute myocardial infarction. *New England Journal of Medicine,* **285**, 190–193.

Hudak, C., Gallo, B. and Lohr, T. (1986) *Critical Care Nursing: a Holistic Approach,* 4th Edn. J.B. Lippincott, Philadelphia.

Weg, J. (1991) Oxygen transport in adult respiratory distress syndrome and other acute circulatory problems: relationship of oxygen delivery and oxygen consumption. *Critical Care Medicine,* **19**, 650–657.

CHAPTER 5

Additional Cardiac Studies

1. INTRODUCTION

Many of the areas outlined in this chapter are still to be evaluated fully and are not accepted as routine assessment. They are included here in order to provide a more comprehensive description of the cardiac function assessments that are currently available.

2. LACTIC ACID BLOOD LEVEL MONITORING

Normal lactic acid blood level = 0.3–2 mmol/l

In impaired tissue perfusion, inadequate oxygenation leads to the anaerobic metabolism of glucose into lactic acid. In normal circumstances this is converted back to glucose in the liver (the Cori cycle). In certain states, increased lactic acid blood levels may occur. Lactic acidaemia results from balance between the body's metabolic needs and tissue oxygen supply.

In the critically ill, a strong positive correlation has been identified between a high blood lactate (greater than 2 mmol/l) and poor patient outcome. Serial measurements of blood lactate levels taken hourly may provide a better prognostic indicator. Levels should be taken serially after treatment has been initiated. A decrease of 10% or greater indicates a positive response to treatment.

3. CONTINUOUS CARDIAC OUTPUT MEASUREMENTS

The bolus thermodilution technique is widely accepted as the standard technique for obtaining CO. However, fluctuations in blood temperature in the PA (e.g. during the respiratory cycle or through operator error) may cause inaccuracies.

Continuous CO uses heat rather than cold as a thermal indicator. Small amounts of heat are given in a 'randomized' on/off sequence from a thermal filament on a modified PA catheter. The thermal filament is located close to the injection port, 13–25 cm from the tip. This has a large surface area (over 10 cm^2) to help heat distribution in the blood. A distal thermistor detects the blood temperature changes in the range of 0.2°C. The thermodilution curve is then calculated by a bedside computer. The computer produces an updated CO every 30–60 sec. Alterations in the thermal noise (e.g. respiration, induced temperature changes) will increase the averaging time.

Continuous CO measurements can also be provided by non-invasive thoracic impedence devices.

4. RIGHT VENTRICULAR FUNCTION STUDIES

Normal values:

Right ventricular end-diastolic volume (RVEDV) = 100–160 ml
Right ventricular end-systolic volume (RVESV) = 50–60 ml
Right ventricular stroke volume (RVSV) = 60–100 ml
Right ventricular ejection fraction (RVEF) = 40–60%

The original Starling function curves used the relationship between SV and end-diastolic volume (preload). The clinical use of PA catheters enables the assessment of the ventricular function curve using the relationship between

SV and end-diastolic pressure. This is based on the assumption that volume = pressure. However, any changes in pressure (e.g. positive end-expiratory pressure, increased pericardial or abdominal pressure) may alter the curve.

Compliance is the relationship between end-diastolic volume and end-diastolic pressure. This relationship is curvilinear, not linear, and therefore volume does not equal pressure. In conditions where there is an increased compliance (e.g. chronic ventricular dilatation, congestive cardiomyopathy), a large change in volume will be associated with a small change in pressure. Where there is a decreased compliance (e.g. myocardial ischaemia, ventricular hypertrophy), a small change in volume will be associated with a large change in pressure.

Techniques available to date to study RV function include echocardiography (which may lack technical quality in critically ill patients) and angiography (impractical to perform serial measurements). With right heart studies there is the facility to assess the ventricular function curve using the original relationship between SV and end-diastolic volume.

In RV failure associated with acute pulmonary hypertension, pulmonary embolism, acute respiratory failure or ARDS, it is now suggested that the thin-walled right ventricle dilates to maintain the SV in the presence of increased RV afterload. This septal shifting into the LV space reduces LV preload and can therefore limit CO. RV perfusion occurs during systole and diastole owing to the lower systolic pressures. In pulmonary hypertension, the increased RV pressures may affect right coronary perfusion. RV dilatation can increase the oxygen demands of the ventricle through increased wall stress contributing to ischaemia. Direct monitoring of RV performance may provide a better guide to fluid or inotropic support in such patients.

To calculate the parameters, a modified PA catheter with proximal (in RV) and distal (in PA) intracardiac electrodes to sense the R wave is used. An additional patient reference is provided either by a further cardiac chest lead or by 'slaving' the patient monitor tracing into the bedside computer. The modified PA catheter can provide data on RVEF, RVESV, RVEDS, SV and HR. By using the R to R interval, CO and right ventricular function values can be calculated. A standard thermodilution CO technique is used to measure CO.

These data can then be used to optimize RV efficiency and the relationship between end-diastolic volume (EDV) and SV through titration of volume and inotropes/vasodilators. The presence of tricuspid regurgitation, intracardiac shunting or tachyarrhythmias will cause errors in the readings by affecting temperature/volume.

5. MEASUREMENTS OF INTRAMUCOSAL pH

Normal intramucosal pH = 7.35–7.45

Changes in gastric intramucosal pH (pHi) may act as an early index of oxygen transport problems. This value can be used as a prognostic indicator, either as a one-off or a trend: a persistently low pHi is associated with higher mortality.

Tissue hypoxia and acidosis decrease splanchnic blood flow and gut perfusion. This increases gut mucosal tissue hydrogen and CO_2 concentration which diffuses until equilibrium is reached between luminal and intramucosal PCO_2. This may promote bacterial translocation from the gut lumen in the septic process.

Measurement of pHi is made by the use of a nasogastric tube with a proximal tonometry balloon. It allows indirect measurement of the PCO_2 in the gut lining. Saline is instilled into the balloon and then withdrawn after a steady state has been achieved (usually after 30–60 min) to obtain PCO_2. An acid–base assessment of the gastric lining pHi can then be calculated with the Henderson–Hasselbach equation. Simultaneous arterial blood must be drawn to determine serum bicarbonate.

6. PRINCIPLES FOR PAEDIATRIC CARDIAC STUDIES

There is less experience with the use of PA catheters and CO studies in paediatrics. For a child, a No. 5 FG (with 0.8 ml balloon) or a No. 4 FG (with 0.35 ml balloon) would be used. Complete obstruction of the right ventricular outflow tract by wedging the balloon may occur during insertion and cause hypoxia and collapse. Rapid deflation and withdrawal of the catheter should resolve this.

As a general guide, typical CO results are:

CVP = 3–5 mmHg
PAWP = 5–8 mmHg
CI   = 3.5–4.5 l/min/m²

Other results are shown in *Table 14*.

PVR is approximately 640–800 dynes/sec/cm⁵ at birth, but by 6–8 weeks of life the PVR has fallen to near the adult values of 80–240 dynes/sec/cm⁵.

Injectate volumes used for CO in paediatrics are smaller than those for adults (3.5–5 ml) to prevent fluid overload. In children, the term 'low CO' is used when the CI is less than 2.2 l/min/m². Untreated haemorrhage or fluid loss/dehydration of 10% or greater will cause a low output state.

Table 14. Results of cardiac studies in paediatrics

Age	CO (l/min)	HR	SV (ml)	SVR (dynes/sec/cm^5)
Newborn	0.8–1.0	135	5	800–1200
6 months	1.0–1.3	120	10	
1 yr	1.3–1.5	115	13	1200–1600
2 yr	1.5–2.0	115	18	
4 yr	2.3–2.75	105	27	
5 yr	2.5–3.0	95	31	1200–2400
8 yr	3.4–3.6	83	42	
10 yr	3.8–4.0	75	50	
15 yr	6.0	70	85	

The development of low CO may quickly deplete glycogen stores, producing hypoglycaemia and further depressing myocardial functioning.

7. RESPIRATORY AND OXYGEN TRANSPORT VARIABLES

There are three important parameters which affect respiratory and oxygen transport measurements:

- cardiac output,
- haemoglobin,
- arterial partial pressure of oxygen.

7.1 Arterial oxygen content (CaO$_2$)

Normal CaO$_2$ = 17–20 ml/dl or 170–200 ml/l of blood

Oxygen is transported in the blood by binding to Hb and, to a small extent, by dissolving directly in the blood. One gram of saturated Hb binds 1.34 ml of oxygen. Every mmHg of arterial oxygen partial pressure corresponds to an oxygen concentration of 0.0031 ml/dl dissolved directly in the blood. The total arterial oxygen content therefore corresponds to the sum of all of these:

$$CaO_2 \ (ml/dl) = (1.34 \times Hb \times SaO_2/100) + (PaO_2 \times 0.0031)$$

Abnormally low readings indicate anaemia or inefficient gas exchange due to pulmonary membrane damage or arteriovenous shunting in the lungs. High readings may indicate that the patient needs reducing levels of oxygen support.

7.2 Venous oxygen content (CvO$_2$)

Normal CvO$_2$ = 120–150 ml/l

CvO$_2$ is the total oxygen content of venous blood. Its calculation is based on principles similar to those used in the formula for CaO$_2$:

CvO$_2$ (ml/dl) = (1.34 × Hb × SvO$_2$/100) + (PvO$_2$ × 0.0031)

Tissues receiving a decreased blood flow will extract oxygen more completely and CvO$_2$ values will be low. This will also be reflected by abnormally high values for the oxygen extraction ratio (O$_2$ER) and arteriovenous difference (AvDO$_2$).

Low readings will be seen in hypovolaemic and cardiogenic shock states where there is reduced or slower blood flow to the peripheries, leading to a greater uptake of O$_2$ by the tissues. CvO$_2$ will rise when tissue oxygen requirements fall, as in hypothyroidism, hypothermia and malnutrition. CvO$_2$ is also high in septic shock, where the rate of blood flow is too fast for unloading and the inability of oxygen uptake at cellular level exacerbates this problem.

7.3 Alveolar–arterial oxygen difference (AaDO$_2$)

Normal AaDo$_2$ = 1.3–2 kPa on 21% O$_2$/room air
= 1.3–6 kPa receiving O$_2$ therapy

This parameter measures the difference in partial pressure of oxygen between the alveoli and the arterial system. It gives an indication of the efficiency of oxygen exchange between the alveoli and pulmonary capillaries. The calculation has to account for barometric pressure (PB) and the partial pressure of water vapour at 37°C (= 47 mmHg). With increasing age, the lungs may not function as effectively and AaDO$_2$ can increase. This effect can be estimated by multiplying the patient's age by 0.4.

AaDO$_2$ (mmHg) = PAO$_2$ – PaO$_2$

where PAO$_2$ = FIO$_2$ × (PB – 47) – PaCO$_2$.

A rise in AaDO$_2$ indicates an increasingly inefficient pulmonary membrane and may warn of impending respiratory failure.

7.4 Arteriovenous oxygen difference (AvDO$_2$)

Normal AvDO$_2$ = 4.2–5 ml/dl

This is a measure comparing arterial and venous oxygen contents. It gives an indication of the amount of oxygen in the systemic capillaries available for tissue consumption. Calculation requires arterial (as part of CaO$_2$) and mixed venous (as part of CvO_2) blood sampling. The difference between the two provides an estimation of tissue perfusion and oxygenation.

$$AvDO_2 \ (ml/dl) = (CaO_2 - CvO_2)$$

High $AvDO_2$ values can indicate increased oxygen extraction at cellular level. This may be as a result of decreased blood flow (e.g. low output state). Values greater than 5.6 ml/dl require urgent attention. Low $AvDO_2$ values demonstrate poor oxygen uptake at cellular level.

7.5 Oxygen availability (O_2AV) and index (O_2AVI)

Normal O_2AV = 800–1200 ml/min
Normal O_2AVI = 550–650 ml/min/m^2

Oxygen availability and index indicate whether the patient's cardiorespiratory system is operating efficiently enough to provide an adequate volume of oxygen to the tissues. Oxygen availability identifies the total amount of oxygen carried in the blood from the heart each minute. The value is calculated by multiplying the oxygen content of the blood by the CO. A multiplication factor of 10 is used to convert decilitres to litres.

$$O_2AV \ (ml/min) \quad = CaO_2 \times CO \times 10$$
$$O_2AVI \ (ml/min/m^2) = CaO_2 \times CI \times 10$$
$$= O_2AV/BSA$$

Oxygen availability falls when oxygen delivery to the tissues is compromised, for example as in cardiogenic shock, with a resultant low CO or pulmonary damage with a low CaO_2. O_2AVI values of less than 400 ml/min/m^2 are a cause for serious concern. A high O_2AV may occur by raising the CO with volume or inotropes/vasodilators or increasing the FiO_2.

7.6 Oxygen consumption (VO_2) and index (VO_2I)

Normal VO_2 = 250–300 ml/min
Normal VO_2I = 115–165 ml/min/m^2

VO_2 reflects the amount of oxygen consumed by the entire body. It is an overall measurement of the body's metabolism: the 'demand' side. It calculates the rate of oxygen consumption over time by multiplying the arteriovenous oxygen difference ($AvDO_2$) by the CO. A multiplication factor of 10 is used to convert decilitres to litres.

$$VO_2 \ (ml/min) \quad = AvDO_2 \times CO \times 10$$
$$VO_2I \ (ml/min/m^2) = AvDO_2 \times CI \times 10$$
$$= VO_2/BSA$$

Oxygen consumption will rise in hyperthyroidism, sepsis, trauma, burns and with the administration of adrenergic drugs. Hypothermia, poor gas exchange and poor tissue perfusion will lower VO_2. In the critically ill, a VO_2I value of 150–200 ml/min/m^2 may be desirable. VO_2I values under 100 ml/min/m^2 are of concern as this can demonstrate that the metabolic needs of the tissues are not being met.

Patient procedures can also affect VO_2 (*Table 15*). This needs to be considered within the patient's care.

Table 15. Patient procedures affecting VO_2

Procedure	Increase (%) in VO_2	Decrease (%) in VO_2
Hypothermia (each °C)	10	
Morphine infusion		9–21
Dressing change	10–25	
ECG	12	
Visitors	22	
Blanket bath	23	
Chest X-ray	22–25	
Anaesthesia		25
Tracheal suctioning	27	
Repositioning	31	
Physiotherapy	20–35	
Nasal intubation	25–40	

7.7 Oxygen delivery (DO_2) and index (DO_2I)

Normal DO_2 = 950–1150 ml/min
Normal DO_2I = 550–650 ml/min/m^2

DO_2 reflects the amount of oxygen delivered to the entire body in ml/min. It gives an indication of the overall function of the circulatory system and the amount of oxygen delivered to the tissues: the 'supply' side. It is calculated by multiplying the arterial oxygen content (CaO_2) by the CO. A multiplication factor of 10 is used to convert decilitres to litres.

$$DO_2 \text{ (ml/min)} = CaO_2 \times CO \times 10$$
$$DO_2I \text{ (ml/min/m}_2) = CaO_2 \times CI \times 10$$
$$= DO_2/BSA$$

A DO_2I below 400 ml/min/m^2 is of concern as this can demonstrate that the metabolic needs of the tissues are not being met. The values of DO_2

and VO_2 must be analysed simultaneously as the adequacy of oxygenation depends on maintaining a balance between oxygen delivery and consumption.

7.8 Oxygen extraction ratio (O_2ER)

Normal O_2ER = 0.24–0.28

O_2ER compares oxygen consumption to oxygen availability (VO_2/O_2AV). It identifies the percentage of delivered oxygen actually consumed by the tissues. The ratio is the fraction of available oxygen that is extracted by the tissues.

$$O_2ER = (CaO_2 - CvO_2)/CaO_2$$

Values greater than 0.30 give cause for concern, and values in excess of 0.35 indicate serious problems. Abnormally high O_2ER values are usually accompanied by high $AvDO_2$.

O_2ER falls when less oxygen is extracted, as in anaemic states, conditions with low tissue O_2 demand (e.g. hypothermia) and in high CO states. O_2ER rises in low CO states when greater oxygen is extracted.

7.9 Percentage arteriovenous shunt (Qs/Qt)

Normal Qs/Qt = 3–5%

Not all blood that returns to the left side of the heart is oxygenated via the lungs. The myocardial wall veins and bronchial arteries drain directly into the left atrium. Mixing of this blood with the oxygenated blood in the left atrium reduces the overall saturation of the systemic arterial blood. In disease, some blood in the pulmonary circulation remains deoxygenated because of flow through poorly ventilated alveoli or through obstructed alveolar capillaries.

The Qs/Qt shunt formula indicates efficiency of the oxygenation system. It is calculated from:

$$Qs/Qt = 100 \times \frac{Hb \times 1.34 \times (1 - (SaO_2/100)) + 0.0031(PAO_2 - PaO_2)}{Hb \times 1.34 \times (1 - (SvO_2/100)) + 0.0031(PAO_2 - PvO_2)}$$

The value is a percentage, but the formula uses measurements of $ml/O_2/dl$ of blood. The more efficient the oxygenation process of the blood, the smaller the Qs/Qt. There are no absolute values to guide treatment, but percentage shunts greater than 20 indicate moderate lung function and reducing/weaning from respiratory support is contraindicated. Shunts greater than 30 indicate severe pulmonary dysfunction.

8. FURTHER READING

Boldt, J. and Menges, T. (1994) Is continuous cardiac output measurement using thermodilution reliable in the critically ill patient? *Critical Care Medicine*, **22**(12), 1913–1918.

Doglio, G., Pusajo, J. *et al.* (1991) Gastric mucosal pH as a prognostic index of mortality in critically ill patients. *Critical Care Medicine*, **19**(8), 1037–1040.

Dorman, B.H. (1992) Use of a combined right ventricular ejection fraction oximetry catheter system for coronary bypass surgery. *Critical Care Medicine*, **20**, 1650.

Gilbert, H.L. (1992) Evaluation of continuous cardiac output in patients undergoing coronary artery surgery. *Anaesthesiology*, **77**, A472.

Hayden, R.A. (1992) What keeps oxygenation on track? *American Journal of Nursing*, December, 32–40.

Hazinski, M. (1984) *Nursing Care of the Critically Ill Child*. C.V. Mosby, St Louis.

Lowery, G. and Trinder, T. (1995) Tonometry in critical illness. *Care of the Critically Ill*, **11** (1), 23–27.

Vincent, J., Dufaye, P. *et al.* (1983) Serial lactate determinations during circulatory shock. *Critical Care Medicine*, **11**(6), 449–451.

Vincent, J. (1990) The measurement of right ventricle ejection fraction. *Intensive Care World*, **7**(3), 133–136.

APPENDIX A

Cardioactive drugs

Three physiological principles need to be considered when supporting circulatory failure. All these parameters can be manipulated to improve cardiac function and maximize haemodynamic stability.

Patient problem	Treatment options
Right ventricular afterload	
Increased	
Chronic obstructive airways	Pulmonary vasodilators (e.g. Aminophylline)
Pulmonary embolism/hypertension	Loop diuretics (e.g. frusemide)
Hypoxaemia	Oxygen therapy
Decreased	
Hypotension	Fluid replacement
Arterial vasodilators	
Left ventricular afterload	
Increased	
Systemic hypertension	Arterial vasodilators (e.g. nitroprusside/hydralazine)
Aortic valve disease	calcium channel blockers (e.g. nifedipine)
Shock states	ACE inhibitors (e.g. captopril/enalapril)
Hypercoagulability	α_1 blockers (e.g. phentolamine/prazosin/labetalol)

continued

	Patient problem	Treatment options
Decreased	Septic/Spinal shock	Arterial vasopressors (e.g. noradrenaline/high dose dopamine)
Preload		
Increased	Congestive cardiac failure	Loop diurectics (e.g. frusemide)
	Fluid overload	Haemofiltration/haemodialysis
Decreased	Hypovolaemia	Replacing circulating volume
	Excessive vasodilation	Administer isotonic crystalloids, colloid, blood
Contractility		
Altered by	Myocardial ischaemia/infarction	Cardiac glycosides (e.g. digoxin)
	Hypoxaemia	Inotropes (e.g. adrenaline, dobutamine)
	Acidosis	Phosphodiesterase inhibitors (e.g. amrinone, milrinone)

INOTROPES

Inotropes increase myocardial **contractility**. They act through stimulation of adrenoceptors of the sympathetic nervous system via the neurotransmitter noradrenaline. They have a half-life of 2–4 minutes. They should not be administered to volume-depleted patients.

Dopamine	*Mode of action:* Stimulates α, β and dopaminergic receptors – dose related.

Clinical effects and use: Increases blood flow to renal, mesenteric, coronary and cerebral areas. High doses – peripheral vasoconstriction with increased peripheral resistance and afterload, with reduced renal blood. Used for cardiac failure and cardiogenic shock.

Dobutamine　　*Mode of action:* Stimulates β_1 receptors and α_1/β_2 receptors.

Clinical effects and use: Increases myocardial contractility with improved CO. Dose-related chronotropic effects related to β_2-mediated vasodilation. Infusion for more than 72 hours may cause down-regulation of myocardial β_1 adrenoceptors resulting in drug tolerance and refractoriness to dobutamine. Used for cardiac failure.

Adrenaline　　*Mode of action:* Stimulates α_1 in high doses; stimulates β_1 in low doses.

Clinical effects and use: Causes vasoconstriction with potential ischaemia. Positive inotropic effect with increased HR, CO and SV. Can induce tachycardias/ tachyarrythmias. Administered as a bolus or infusion. Half-life of 1–2 minutes. Used for low output states.

PRACTICE POINT

Only dobutamine can be administered peripherally if central venous access is not available.

Noradrenaline　　*Mode of action:* Stimulates α receptors and β_1 receptors.

Clinical effects and use: Increases SVR. Positive inotropic action and enhanced myocardial contractility and increasing HR, CO, SV and myocardial oxygen consumption. Constriction of all arterial vascular beds. Used for septic shock to increase SVR.

> **PRACTICE POINT**
> For cardiac arrest use 1 mg/10 ml (1:10 000). For continuous infusion use 10 mg/10 ml (1:1000) via a central venous access with a dedicated lumen. Induced hyperglycaemia may require an insulin infusion due to glucose production.

Isoprenaline *Mode of action:* Stimulates β receptors.
Clinical effects and use: Positive chronotropic effect and potent pulmonary vasodilator. Use for bradycardia and complete heart block, right-sided heart failure with elevated PVR.

VASODILATORS

Vasodilators reduce **afterload** by reducing systemic or pulmonary vascular resistance. This lowers the impedance to ventricular ejection and therefore increases CO. The resultant decrease in ventricular wall tension and ventricle end-diastolic volumes reduces ventricular oxygen requirements. They have a half-life of 2–4 minutes.

Glyceryl trinitrate *Mode of action:* Increases venous capacitance. Predominant venodilator.
Clinical effects and use: Reduces venous return. Reduces afterload. Used for hypertension, ischaemic heart disease.

Sodium nitroprusside *Mode of action:* Mixed arteriolar and venous dilator.
Clinical effects and use: Decreases afterload. Used for hypertension.

> **PRACTICE POINT**
> Administration and monitoring practices with this drug should follow manufacturer's recommendations.

Nitric oxide *Mode of action:* Pulmonary smooth muscle vasodilation.
Clinical effects and use: Short acting, selective pulmonary vasodilator. Only dilates ventilated areas of lung. Rapidly bound to haemoglobin to form methaemoglobin. Administered with inspired gas on ventilated patient. Used for pulmonary hypertension in adults and paediatrics/ neonates.

> **PRACTICE POINT**
> Attention to cardiovascular and respiratory parameters should occur during administration and slow weaning of this drug.

INODILATORS

Dopexamine   *Mode of action:* Stimulates β_2 receptors. Adrenergic agent.
Clinical effects and use: Decreases systemic and pulmonary vascular resistance. Combined inotrope and vasodilatory effects – inodilator. Increases blood flow to hepatic, splanchnic and renal vascular beds. Used for cardiac failure, post-abdominal surgery.

Milrinone   *Mode of action:* Phosphodiesterase inhibitor. Increases cAMP. Increases calcium entry into cells.
Clinical effects and use: Vasodilation and improved myocardial contractility. Reduces PAWP and increases LVSWI and maintains oxygen supply/demand ratio. Used for end-stage congestive cardiac failure, cardiogenic shock.

VOLUME REPLACEMENT

The major goal of fluid therapy is to create an adequate **preload** which increases SV and therefore CO. When fluid adminstration is no longer suffi-cient to maintain a blood pressure adequate for tissue perfusion, vasopressor and/or inotropic support are indicated.

> **PRACTICE POINT**
> Large transfusions of citrated blood may cause a decrease in serum calcium; 10 ml of 10% calcium gluconate (contains 90 mg elemental calcium) can provide restoration and create a positive inotropic action.

Whole blood   *Constituents:* Restores blood volume and Hb.
Clinical use: Increases the O_2 carrying capacity of the blood.

Red blood cells   *Constituents:* Contain plasma, few leukocytes and plate-lets.
Clinical use: Increases haematocrit in patients below 0.35%.

Platelets

Constituents: Contain platelets, some plasma and lymphocytes.
Clinical use: Control bleeding and maintain normal platelet count. If platelet concentration falls below 20 000 units, then transfusion is recommended.

Fresh frozen plasma

Constituents: Contains all plasma proteins, clotting factors (contains no platelets, red or white blood cells).
Clinical use: Restores clotting factors, acts as a plasma volume expander.

PRACTICE POINT

Once thawed must be administered within 2 hours to prevent deterioration of clotting factors V and VIII.

Albumin

Constituents: Contains no blood-clotting properties. Available in 4.5%/20% in a solution. Prepared from whole blood.
Clinical use: Rapid plasma volume expander. Used to treat hypoalbuminaemia.

Hetastarch

Constituents: Hydroxyethyl starch. Available in 6%/10% in a solution of isotonic saline.
Clinical use: Volume expander with a long half-life (up to 36 hours). Maximal infusion in acute haemorrhage – 20 l/kg/h. Hyperamylasaemia may occur due to slow elimination.

Gelofusin
Haemaccel

Constituents: Chemically modified gelatins.
Clinical use: Immediate short-acting plasma expanders.

Hartmann's

Constituents: 0.6% sodium chloride with electrolytes and buffers.
Clinical use: Replaces circulatory volume and buffers acidosis.

PRACTICE POINT

Hartmann's contains 27 meq/l lactate – use with caution in patients unable to tolerate metabolic acid load (e.g. diabetics and shocked patients).

APPENDIX B

Cardiac output studies and vital signs

Calculations for derived cardiac output study parameters

MAP	$= \dfrac{\text{systolic BP} + 2 \, (\text{diastolic BP})}{3}$
CI	$= \dfrac{\text{CO}}{\text{BSA}}$
SVR	$= \dfrac{(\text{MAP} - \text{RA}) \times 79.96}{\text{CO}}$
PVR	$= \dfrac{(\text{MPAP} - \text{PWP}) \times 79.96}{\text{CO}}$
SV	$= \dfrac{\text{CO} \times 100}{\text{HR}}$
LCWI	$= \dfrac{\text{MAP} \times \text{CO} \times 0.0136}{\text{BSA}}$
LVSWI	$= \dfrac{\text{MAP} \times \text{SV} \times 0.0136}{\text{BSA}}$
RCWI	$= \dfrac{\text{MPAP} \times \text{CO} \times 0.0136}{\text{BSA}}$
RVSWI	$= \dfrac{\text{MPAP} \times \text{SV} \times 0.0136}{\text{BSA}}$

Values for cardiac output study paramaters – adults

Heart rate	HR	60–100 beats/min
Arterial blood pressure	BP	100–140 mmHg
		60–90
Mean arterial pressure	MAP	80–95 mmHg
Right atrial pressure	RAP	2–10 mmHg
Pulmonary artery pressure	PAP	15–25 mmHg
		8–15
Mean Pulmonary pressure	MPAP	10–20 mmHg
Pulmonary wedge pressure	PWP	6–12 mmHg
Cardiac output	CO	4–8 l/min
Cardiac index	CI	2.5–4 l/min/m^2
Systemic vascular resistance	SVR	900–1600 dynes/sec/cm^5
Pulmonary vascular resistance	PVR	20–120 dynes/sec/cm^5
Stroke volume	SV	60–100ml/beat
Left cardiac work index	LCWI	3.4–4.2 kg/m/m^2
Left ventricular stroke work index	LVSWI	50–62 g/m/m^2
Right cardiac work index	RCWI	0.54–0.66 kg/m/m^2
Right ventricular stroke work index	RVSWI	7.9–9.7 g/m/m^2
Mixed venous oxygen saturation	SvO$_2$	60–80%

Vital signs for paediatrics and neonates – normal values

Age (years)	Heart rate (beats/min)	BP (Systolic) (mmHg)	Respirations (/min)
Neonate	120–160	45–65	30–60
2–5	120–140	80–90	20–30
5–12	80–100	90–110	15–20
Adolescents	60–90	95–140	12–16

Estimating circulating blood volume – ml/kg

Neonates	85–90
2–5 years	75–80
5–12 years	70–75
Adults	65–70

Urine output – ml/kg/h

0–2 years	2.0 ml
2–12 years	1.0 ml
Adults	0.5 ml

APPENDIX C

Additional information

These data have been taken from M.J. Parr and T.M. Craft (1994) *Resuscitation: key data,* 2nd Edn. BIOS Scientific Publishers, Oxford.

COAGULATION

Platelet count ($\times 10^9$/l)	150–400
Bleeding time (min)	<7
Prothrombin time (sec)	11.5–15
Activated partial thromboplastin time (sec)	25–37
Thombin time (sec)	10
Fibrinogen (g/l)	2–4.5
FDPs (mg/l)	<10

BIOCHEMISTRY

	Neonate	Child	Adult
Na (mmol/l)	130–145	132–145	133–143
K (mmol/l)	4.0–7.0	3.5–5.5	3.6–4.6Cl
Cl (mmol/l)	95–110	95–110	95–105
Cr (μmol/l)	28–60	30–80	60–100
Urea (mmol/l)	1.0–5.0	2.5–6.5	3–7
Mg (mmol/l)	0.6–1.0	0.6–1.0	0.7–1
Ca (mmol/l)	1.8–2.8	2.15–2.7	2.25–2.7
Phosphate (mmol/l)	1.3–3.0	1.0–1.8	0.85–1.4
Billirubin (μmol/l)	<200	<15	<17
Alkaline phosphate (U/l)	150–600	250–1000	21–120
AST (U/l)	<100	<50	6–35
Total protein (g/l)	45–75	60–80	62–80
Albumin (g/l)	24–48	30–50	35–55
Globulin (g/l)	20–30	20–30	22–36

BLOOD GASES

Arterial

pH	7.34–7.46
PaO_2 [kPa (mmHg)]	10–13.3 (75–100)
$PaCO_2$ [kPa(mmHg)]	4.4–6.1 (33–46)
Actual bicarbonate (mmol/l	22–26
Standard bicarbonate (mmol/l)	22–26
Base excess	±2
Oxygen saturation	0.96–1.0

Mixed Venous

pH	7.32–7.42
PaO_2 [kPa(mmHg)]	4.96–5.6 (36–42)
$PaCO_2$ [kPa(mmHg)]	5.3–6.9 (40–52)
Oxygen saturation	0.78–0.8

Conversion factors

1 mmHg = 133.3 Pa = 1.36 cmH_2O = 1.25 cm blood
100 mmHg = 13.3 kPa
760 mmHg = 101.3 kPa
1 kPa = 7.5 mmHg = 10.2 cmH_2O
1 mmH_2O = 0.073 mmHg
100 kPa = 15 psi
1 atm = 1 Bar = 101.3 kPa = 1033 cmH_2O

Coventry University

ANTIARRHYTHMIC DRUG DOSES

Adenosine: by rapid i.v. injection	3 mg
2nd dose (if required)	6 mg
3rd dose (if required)	12 mg
Further dosage not recommended	

Amiodarone: over 20–120 min (via	5 mg/kg
central vein) max. dose in 24 h	1.2 g

Bretylium: over 8–10 min repeated after	5–10 mg/kg
1–2 h to a total dosage of	30 mg/kg

Digoxin: initial i.v. dose over >1 h   0.75–1 mg

Esmolol: initial i.v. dose over 1 min	500 µg/kg
followed by infusion for 4 min of	50 µg/kg/min

The loading dose may then be repeated
and the maintenance infusion rate doubled
if the response is inadequate.

Lignocaine: initial slow bolus	100 mg
followed by infusion of	2–4 mg/min

Verapamil: by slow bolus   5–10 mg

INFUSION DRUG DOSES

Dopamine	2–15 µg/kg/min
Dobutamine	2–20 µg/kg/min
Adrenaline	0.01–0.5 µg/kg/min
Noradrenaline	0.01–0.5 µg/kg/min
Isoprenaline	0.5–10 µg/min
Aminophylline: loading dose	5 mg/kg
(over 20 min) followed by	500 µg/kg/h

Nitroprusside: initial rate	0.3–1 µg/kg/min
Usual dose range	0.5–6 µg/kg/min
Maximum dose	8 µg/kg/min

Glyceryl trinitrate   10–200/µg/min

Note:
These doses are the usual ranges and do not preclude the use of an initial bolus or much higher infusion doses in exceptional circumstances.

Index

Coventry University

ORDERING DETAILS

Main address for orders

BIOS Scientific Publishers Ltd
9 Newtec Place, Magdalen Road,
Oxford OX4 1RE, UK
Tel: +44 1865 726286
Fax: +44 1865 246823

Australia and New Zealand
DA Information Services
648 Whitehorse Road, Mitcham, Victoria 3132, Australia
Tel: (03) 9210 7777
Fax: (03) 9210 7788

India
Viva Books Private Ltd
4325/3 Ansari Road, Daryaganj, New Delhi 110 002, India
Tel: 11 3283121
Fax: 11 3267224

Singapore and South East Asia
(Brunei, Hong Kong, Indonesia, Korea, Malaysia, the Philippines,
Singapore, Taiwan, and Thailand)
Toppan Company (S) PTE Ltd
38 Liu Fang Road, Jurong, Singapore 2262
Tel: (265) 6666
Fax: (261) 7875

USA and Canada
BIOS Scientific Publishers
PO Box 605, Herndon, VA 20172-0605, USA
Tel: (703) 661 1500
Fax: (703) 661 1501

Payment can be made by cheque or credit card (Visa/Mastercard, quoting number and expiry date). Alternatively, a *pro forma* invoice can be sent.

Prepaid orders must include £2.50/US$5.00 to cover postage and packing (two or more books sent post free)